Praise & Feedback

With the rise of chemical contamination, genetic manipulation, and corporate control of our food supply, nutritional literacy has become an essential survival skill. And there is no better resource to educate oneself than Evita Ochel's smart, no-nonsense, easy-to-read guide to healthy eating. Healing & Prevention Through Nutrition teaches us about the relationships between diet and disease and how a lifestyle that incorporates natural, whole, unprocessed foods is the best medicine. Highly recommended!

—Larry Malerba, DO, holistic physician and author of *Green Medicine* and *Metaphysics & Medicine,* SpiritScienceHealing.com

This is what REAL eating is all about. Finally a common-sense book to enlighten and inspire everyone towards making better food choices. Seeing beyond all the junk that masquerades as 'food' nowadays, you will understand the TRUTH of the cause of disease and then realize the power to ultimately control your health by what goes into your body. And to all the dieters out there...ditch every gimmick you've tried and toss the diet books. A must-read for anyone who wants to live the life that they have imagined—full of health and VITALITY.

—Colette Szalay, DC, chiropractic doctor, Ontario, Canada

It has never been more important to understand the connection between the foods you put into your mouth and your overall health. Diabetes, obesity, heart disease and countless other diseases are rampant in our modern world. What do these diseases have in common? They are, in large part, the result of the food choices you make every day. Evita Ochel's *Healing & Prevention Through Nutrition* is a book with a powerful nutritional punch. Evita's advice of low-calorie, high nutrition, plant-based, and low processed food is exactly what you need to get yourself on track to a healthier and more energetic you.

—Scott Olson, ND, naturopathic doctor and author of *Sugarettes,* OlsonND.com

Evita does a remarkable job of having a conversation about health, not a dissertation. Evita shows us that healthy eating is not about food groups and daily allowances, it's about clean eating and re-acknowledging the human relationship we have with food. *Healing & Prevention Through Nutrition* offers no agenda other than to provide practical nutrition tips and advice, and to remind us that health is our most valuable asset.

—Alexander J. Rinehart, MS, DC, CCN, clinical nutritionist
and chiropractor, DrAlexRinehart.com

Evita's lifelong commitment and passion for natural health and wellness resonates in her words and every action in her life. In this book, Evita returns the power of personal health back where it belongs—to you! With so much misinformation out there, this material finally offers honest, easy and detailed info to help you understand the right choices to make for any healthy goal— weight loss, healing foods, better energy, longevity. A must-have gift for anyone seriously interested in healing their body and making the right nutritional choices for themselves and their family for life!

—Unity J. Schmidt, energy healer and life path guide, HealingWithUnity.com

Healing and Prevention Through Nutrition is one of the best natural nutrition resources I have read. It teaches and reminds you of how to maintain health and prevent disease through food. Not only is it informative, easy to understand, and well laid out, but it is also truly inspirational. Evita makes eating for optimal health achievable for anyone and everyone and that's what makes this book a must-read!

—Allison Jorgens, BSc., P.H.Ec., food labels specialist
and author of *Read It With A Grain of Salt*

Healing & Prevention Through Nutrition

Second Edition • Fully Revised and Expanded

A Holistic Approach to Eating and Living for
Optimal Health, Weight, and Wellness

Evita Ochel

Foreword by
Elaine R. Ferguson, MD

MATRIX
FUSIONS

For information, address:
Matrix Fusions
4936 Yonge Street, Suite #722
Toronto, ON, M2N 6S3
Web: www.matrixfusions.com
Email: info@matrixfusions.com

To contact the author directly, visit: www.evitaochel.com

Originally published in 2011. Second edition published 2014.

ISBN-13: 978-0-9939645-0-3
ISBN-10: 0993964508

Photography, cover and interior design by Matrix Fusions

On the cover: An arrangement of spinach, strawberries, and almonds, representing the foundation of nutrition for healing and prevention, where the core of our diets are based on vegetables, especially leafy greens, along with fruits and plant seeds, which include all nuts, seeds, beans, lentils, and grains.

A Dedication for You

This book is dedicated to all who have a sincere interest in being fully alive and living to the highest potential of their health and wellbeing.

For all of you who are choosing to take full accountability and responsibility for your health, *may all the right resources always arrive right when you need them.*

For all of you who are embracing the power of real food and nutrition, *may you always have access to good, natural, wholesome food.*

For all of you who are learning that we are not enslaved by our genes, *may you actively continue to create the most beneficial environment for the wellbeing of your mind and body.*

For all of you who understand that pharmaceuticals and invasive medical procedures should be the exception rather than the norm, *may you mindfully explore the multitude of holistic modalities for healing and prevention.*

For all of you who are recognizing and awakening to the natural healing ability of the body, *may you consciously support your body with all it needs to function optimally, leaving out all that harms.*

For all of you who are leading the way by changing conditioned habits into conscious choices, changing our society one person, one family at a time, *may you enjoy the benefits of optimal health and longevity.*

Contents

Foreword

Across the globe today, the greatest threat to the health and wellbeing of billions of people living in the industrialized world resides primarily in what we eat: the adulterated, over-processed, nutrient-depleted, pesticide-rich, and genetically-modified substances masquerading as food. This is the international public health emergency that must be addressed by those at risk. We cannot rely on anything to save us from the chronic diseases these so-called foods cause, such as cancer, diabetes, heart disease, depression, arthritis, and many, many more.

The body's ability to heal itself is remarkably vast, and when we give it what it needs, it will provide us with the good health we desire, and deserve. We are what we eat, and when we consume the foods Mother Nature intended for us to consume, we are nourished, healed, and provided with the fuel that makes not only our bodies healthy, but our emotions as well. Quite simply, good nutrition is the foundation of the healthy cellular environment that is needed to create optimal health and wellbeing.

I have witnessed thousands of times the power appropriate nutritional interventions play in the reversal of diseases, and the creation of health. This is primarily due to the subclinical nutrient deficiencies that are rampant in the United States. In addition to the aforementioned reliance on highly processed foods, the nutrient quality of foods has significantly diminished over the past fifty years.

Healing & Prevention Through Nutrition is a clarion call to nutritional and health empowerment. Evita is indeed a nutritional troubadour providing a laser-sharp guidance light of substantive evidence-based information, common sense, and ancient truths. While one may ask if there is a need for another book

1

on nutrition, this book, in its elegant simplicity provides guidance, information, and a pathway to greater foundational health and wellbeing.

Evita's depth and breadth of knowledge provides a comprehensive, yet succinct clarification of the confusion surrounding nutritional, dietary, and dieting myths that have led to unnecessary public scrutiny and subversion of the accurate notion of good nutrition, and what the human body needs to function properly in the public arena. She successfully unravels the vast body of misinformation and misunderstanding, and sets the reader on the path to full-bodied understanding.

She also emphasizes the critical importance of a holistic approach not only to nutrition, but to health as well. Yes, nutrition is the foundation, but so is taking care of your mind and spirit. Like optimal health, disease is a dynamic process involving the entire body, even if only one organ system is seemingly affected. Optimal health cannot be achieved through nutrition alone, or treating physical symptoms while ignoring the underlying psychological and emotional issues that are now understood to cause illness. To achieve a balanced state of health in an ongoing manner and develop an effective treatment plan for anything that ails the body, it must be inclusive and take physical, emotional, and psychological factors into consideration.

This book will inform you, enlighten you, and empower you with the information and inspiration to take charge of your health and wellbeing through a holistic approach to optimal nutrition and living.

Thank you Evita for your magnificent contribution.

Elaine R. Ferguson, MD
Author of *Superhealing: Engaging Your Mind, Body, and Spirit to Create Optimal Health and Well-Being*

Introduction

Our current human society has come to a very interesting time, a time when we have lost touch with one of the most basic abilities we have as an animal species living on this planet: knowing how to feed ourselves properly.

There is good news though. Slowly but surely, the tables are turning. Unfortunately, this is not happening quickly enough for many who continue to endure the pain, suffering, and decreased quality of life associated with poor health. A large proportion of us still do not give the process of food acquisition, cooking, or eating the proper attention it deserves, apart from whether it will satisfy our taste buds and time constraints. All too often, we enter the grocery store and grab something from the endless variety of products, merely out of habit or routine. Cooking nowadays is more comprised of opening prepackaged food than actually preparing the food oneself. Plus, there is always the all-too-convenient option to stop at a local fast food restaurant to grab breakfast, lunch, or dinner.

All this would have been fine, perhaps, if what we were getting from the grocery stores and restaurants was real, quality food—nutrition to keep us healthy, nourished, and balanced, to heal and protect us from states of disease. Unfortunately, this is not the case. The vast majority of the food around us is not worthy of being called food, as it is does the exact opposite of what food should do in our bodies. This is where we face one of our biggest challenges as consumers. We must be conscious enough to see past the illusion that has been placed before us, this thing called *food*, and return to food's real, natural, and health-promoting origins.

You have made a decision to pick up this book, so I imagine that you already have your own personal motivation for taking your food choices seriously.

Perhaps it is dealing with your present health, to address healing or your future health, to address prevention, or any combination of these. Whether it is your weight, energy level, or overall wellbeing, the quality of nutrition will play a major role, and have a direct influence. Whatever your personal needs may be, I want to give you some more motivation for your journey, to validate that you have made the right choice and encourage you to continue moving in this positive, healthy direction.

"Cancer Is a Preventable Disease that Requires Major Lifestyle Changes," reads the title of a 2008 expert review published in the Pharmaceutical Research Journal.[1] For just a moment, consider the implications of this statement alone. How many people do you know who live with the idea that cancer is random, unpredictable, unpreventable, or genetic? Perhaps you believe this yourself. Next, consider the source of this information. It does not come from a holistic, alternative, or natural health-oriented source; if it did, you might not find such a statement all that surprising. Rather, this is taken from a team of 8 science experts who examined 120 research studies, with the results published in an official journal of the American Association of Pharmaceutical Scientists. In summary, the report explains that only 5 to 10 percent of all cancer cases can be attributed to genetic defects, whereas the remaining 90 to 95 percent are environment and lifestyle directed. For the purpose of our discussion, 30 to 35 percent of cancers can be attributed specifically to diet, the remainder to factors like tobacco, alcohol, environmental toxins, stress, obesity, and physical inactivity. What does this mean? Simple: You and I have a huge say in increasing or decreasing our risk of cancer based on our daily choices.

This revelation does not apply to cancer alone. There is much information like that above, all with ample supporting evidence, for the majority of diseases and health conditions: heart disease, Type 2 diabetes, osteoporosis, Alzheimer's, hormonal and digestive imbalances, common viral and bacterial infections, and more. What you eat (or don't eat) will play an integral role in your chances of getting sick. Not only that, but if you do get sick, a mounting body of evidence from both conventional and holistic practitioners alike reflects the effectiveness of diet as a healing tool, whether alone or in conjunction with another therapy. One of our greatest health challenges in modern society is not whether we can prevent or heal an illness; rather, it is how to get this vital information to the public and have it be applied. As the saying goes, "We can lead a horse to water, but we cannot make it drink."

Getting the information out there should not be a problem, especially in our technologically-driven age of readily available information, where one click connects us to pretty much anything we want to know. Nevertheless, this is our first obstacle for four main reasons. First, there is a lot of noise and distraction out there, too much misinformation polluting the quality information. Second, much of the quality information seems to be contradictory in nature. Third, and part of why the first two problems exist to begin with, are corporate and independent financial agendas, which obscure and spin information in their favor or blatantly try to suppress it. Last, we cannot force anyone to seek the information, even when it is available, nor can we force them to actually apply it; as already stated, this is our most stifling limitation.

Amidst our modern, industrialized, processed landscape, healthy eating has become a challenge. Between the multitude of diet fads, studies, headlines, and nutrition experts popping up each day, it is hard to know who can be trusted or what can be believed. Many feel it is only possible to eat healthy and correctly when one comes from the right socioeconomic or educational background. Others believe a degree in nutrition is required if one is to have any feasible understanding of nutrition. This could not be farther from the truth. In fact, from a general perspective, we all harbor an innate knowledge of how to feed ourselves properly. Although some argue that we have lost this instinct completely, I feel it has simply been misplaced, that we have forgotten or chosen to ignore what is elementary to us. Nonetheless, when we make a choice to tap into that innate ability, we can make a healthy diet work on any budget or with any educational level.

Think about this: Have you ever seen an overweight wild animal? Whether a squirrel, a bird, a fish or elephant, every wild creature knows how to feed itself, maintain its natural size, and, for the most part, avert disease. Science today knows that cancer incidence rates, like most other lifestyle disease occurrences, are rare in nature to this day, just as they were in earlier humans.[2] Other than for the human animal, which is still considered by the majority to be the most intelligent, none start their day consumed by thoughts of what they should eat, how many calories they should consume, what is good for them, or what amount of nutrients they need. Typically, mother animals teach their offspring what to eat, yet each animal naturally self-moderates with respect to food quantity. The same cannot be said today for humans or the animals in their care, such as our cats and dogs. Our parents are our first (and often main) authorities when it comes to food choices; unfortunately, in the past few generations, what has been modeled and offered to children, resulting in lifelong habits, has gotten progressively worse. A large part of this still comes down to personal choice, but there are two main areas that have made the choices more difficult: the industrialization of our food supply and our increasingly unnatural lifestyles. Therefore, it comes as no surprise that our health and weight statistics have also come to reflect this pattern; they, too, are growing progressively worse.

According to the World Health Organization (WHO), as of 2011, three out of five people (60 percent) worldwide die from lifestyle-related diseases: cancer, diabetes, cardiovascular, and chronic respiratory disease.[3] Four of the most common lifestyle risk factors for these and other diseases continue to be cited: tobacco and/or alcohol use, physical inactivity, and poor diet. Additionally, obesity and weight problems are at unprecedented levels, and these are often the sole precursors for lifestyle diseases. Various sources estimate that anywhere from two-thirds to three-quarters of the North American population is overweight today.

Our downward health and nutrition spiral has been analyzed in many interesting ways, and there are even those of us who think we are doing quite well. Some argue that we live longer than ever before and that earlier humans were not prone to the many chronic diseases we have due to their shorter lifespan. Such an analysis doesn't seem to take into consideration that cancer and other lifestyle diseases are increasingly present in younger people in our population. In fact, our children are being born with, predisposed to, or diagnosed with all sorts of previously rare conditions at alarming rates. Second, we cannot entirely discount that earlier human civilizations did not live as long. This is a commonly held assumption, but it is, in no way, a proven fact across all cultures and timelines. Our perceived "long" lifespan is also very artificial and poor in quality. Most people are kept alive via pharmaceutical, surgical, and other medical means; this is not a natural or quality longevity by any means, and it should not be considered part of one's natural lifespan. It is also important to note here that we do not have to choose between a short lifespan of good quality and a long lifespan of poor quality. We have a third choice, and this is where healing and prevention through nutrition plays a monumental role.

When we begin to connect the dots, we start to see that if and when animals are left to their own devices, in their natural environment, they know perfectly well how to both survive and thrive. They know what to eat, how much to eat, how much movement is necessary, and what substances to avoid. When it comes to us, however, we appear to have been hypnotized by our processed and often very unnatural modern way of life. Our often naïve, nonchalant thinking has infiltrated every aspect of our being and numbed our ability to discern what is best for us, despite our innate wisdom.

The good news is that we are finding our way back home. An increasing number of people each day—people like you and me—are reawakening our sense of knowing how to eat and what to eat for optimal functioning of the human body. As we actively expand our consciousness, we transcend the unconscious, robotic, hypnotic states we have allowed ourselves to live in for far too long. Today, we are taking back our health. We are taking back our quality of life and embracing a healthier balance between modern convenience and our natural state of being.

The purpose of this book is not to feature or reveal some new diet or way of eating. In fact, depending on your personal health journey thus far, you may find few grand revelations in these pages. First and foremost, it is my intention to help you remember your innate potential and inspire you to apply it in your daily life. The modern nutrition landscape may be confusing and even flat out grim-looking at times, but this book will greatly simplify things so you can navigate through it with ease and clarity. It will help you remember what real food is, what your body truly needs, and that your body's natural state is a state of health, not one of disease and illness.

This book is also meant to serve as a resource of the healthiest, most basic and sustainable way to feed ourselves and our families—a method that will prevent illness, support the body's natural healing ability, and maintain an optimal state of health and wellbeing. It is meant to give you a guiding nudge to find your way back home.

We cannot deny that food plays a major role in our lives, and it has since the beginning of time. In every culture, it is often the foundation of celebrations and used to commemorate all sorts of occasions. It is part of our gift-giving and personal enjoyment. We can still have all that, and as we pursue optimal eating, we must be aware that we are not trying to negate food's multidimensional purpose. We simply need to alter our approach and take into conscious consideration some essential fundamentals. We must also respect what we have learned on this planet thus far about how our bodies function and the role our food choices play in the creation of our health or lack thereof. When we realize the potential of whole, natural food, we will become aware that healthy and delicious really do go hand in hand. In doing so, we will be empowered to make enjoyable choices that benefit our short and long term wellbeing.

In pursuing nutritional excellence, our main focus is always on quality. While adding more years to our lives would be nice (optimal nutrition is linked to increased longevity, after all), it is ultimately about increasing the quality of our lives, from the very beginning right through to the very end. Your journey will be very personal, based on how far you are willing to go in your personal evolution at any given time to live up to the highest potential of your being. Taking this journey is not about trying to please others, to fit in with the status quo, or to be a passive follower. Rather, it is about being true to yourself, becoming a leader and creating a healthier society, one person at a time. It is about standing up for what is important to you and what you value the most. It is about being the change you wish to see.

The success of your journey into optimal health, where you will take advantage of your body's natural healing ability and the power of food, will depend a lot on your personal level of confidence, self-love, and self-respect. It will require a great deal of courage, perseverance, and discipline at first, but these are all welcome when we consider what is at stake. Before you know it, your shift in perspective about food and health will become second nature to you, making your actions feel natural, joyous, and effortless. This holistic journey will not only redefine food for you, but it will also force you to confront your relationship with food and with yourself. It will force you to examine the

8

choices you make and the reasons behind them. It will be illuminating and liberating as you step into a more conscious, more empowered way of living. It will help you grow in awareness, expand your consciousness, and evolve to be in alignment with both your body's and our planet's needs and modern challenges. It will align you with the most beneficial way of living for today's times and tomorrow's sustainability. With all this in mind, let's begin the journey into optimal health using the most fundamental tool: our food!

PART 1
How to Eat for Optimal Health

When it comes to eating right and exercising, there is no,
"I'll start tomorrow." Tomorrow is disease.

— Terri Guillemets

CHAPTER 1
Understanding the Basics of Food

Once we decide to get on track and get serious about our health, prevent future states of disease, and heal any existing conditions, we begin to expand our awareness of nutrition by gathering resources on healthy eating. I wish I could tell you this is the fun and easy part, but you probably already realize that it can, on the contrary, be the most confusing and challenging part. Why? Because it seems wherever you look, there is contradictory information about health and nutrition. One day, low carb is in; the next day, it's all about high carb. One day, a particular food item is linked with helping a certain condition; by that very afternoon, it might be linked to causing some other condition. Catchy news headlines about nutrition are created to get our attention but rarely tell the complete or accurate story. Oftentimes, even the most respected and trusted health experts cannot agree on one common approach. In this chapter, we will explore and clarify some reasons why this is so and further address it in our last chapter, when we talk about the role of the mind.

First, our journey begins with understanding the basics of how food can work for or against us. Albert Einstein once said, "Reality is merely an illusion, albeit a very persistent one." With this wisdom in mind, we can begin to expand our perception and realize that the "reality" placed before us today when it comes to food and health is nothing more than a clever illusion. It has been successful at keeping so many of us disempowered, lost, and confused when it comes to our food choices and the state of our health. We have been led to believe that chemically altered substances are adequate food choices, that animal products are the foundation of a good diet, that our genes govern our health, and that bodies stricken by illness are helpless without pharmaceutical intervention. When we look a little deeper, we begin to see that the main source of the nutrition confusion out there has much to do with processed foods and those manufactured and sold with big financial ties to various corporations and organizations. We hear and learn what each special interest group or business wants us to hear and learn. Naturally, each party will represent their product in the best light, and they often play on people's fears and emotions. This may result in desirable outcomes for them and their bottom lines, but it leaves us confused. Out of desperation, most of us give up and follow the path of convenience, our taste buds, or the latest fad without consciously considering what our bodies need or the consequences of our actions.

If we are interested in healing and prevention, as well as enjoying optimal weight and wellbeing, we must realize the big problem with the way most people eat today and why we cannot continue down this path. Diets high in processed foods, animal foods, and calories—the way most people in industrialized nations eat today—result in five main problems:

1. Inflammation

2. Oxidative stress / Free radical damage

3. Toxicity

4. Biochemical imbalance

5. Excess weight

Most science and medical professionals today agree that inflammation is at the physical root of nearly every disease. Inflammation is a protective immune system response that tries to repair damage to any afflicted area. It is expressed by capillary enlargement and a surge of white blood cells, resulting in heat, pain, redness, swelling and disturbed normal function within that area. It begins as a protective response, but when it turns chronic, it becomes destructive rather than constructive. Frequent recurrence results in a chronically overactive immune system that keeps attacking our cells, tissues, and organs, yielding disease. The kind of inflammation we are talking about here results from foods that have inflammatory effects on our cells, tissues, and organs.

Oxidative stress results from an imbalance between reactive oxygen species (i.e. free radicals) and antioxidants that are used to detoxify them and repair the damage caused by them. The damaging molecules come from a variety of sources in our environment, namely our food, water, and air. They commonly cause chain reactions that can result in various harm, like DNA damage and even the death of cells. Just like with inflammation, oxidative stress is considered one of the leading causes of most of the chronic diseases that impact us today. Aside from having a direct connection to the manifestation of diseases like cancer, heart disease, and Alzheimer's, it is also linked to premature or accelerated aging. Oxidative stress can be minimized or even eliminated by reducing the amount of damaging substances coming in and increasing the amount of antioxidants.

The toxic nature of our modern world, where harmful chemicals are not only found in our food, water, and air but also in our personal care products, clothes, cars, and homes, has put a huge stress on our bodies. According to Bruce Lourie and Rick Smith, leading Canadian environmental experts and authors of the book *Toxin Toxout*, there are over 80,000 synthetic chemicals in use in commerce today. Most of these have not been adequately tested for safety, and we are seeing an increasing amount of health and weight problems directly associated with them. Where our food is concerned, pesticides are one of the key areas of concern, as are various additives (preservatives, artificial sweeteners, colors, and flavors). If toxins are water-soluble, they may be readily and regularly eliminated by the body, but they can still cause considerable damage during their time spent within us. Their elimination is also greatly dependent on the proper functioning of our detoxification organs (liver, kidneys, intestines, etc.); if these are sluggish, there is even more cause for concern, because the chemicals will overstay their welcome, possibly causing harm all the while. Fat-soluble toxins like *bisphenol A* (BPA) (found in some plastics and cans used to package our food) or *triclosan* (found in antibacterial soaps and products) may, in some cases, be metabolized and excreted out of the body, but they typically tend to accumulate, specifically in our fat cells. Many toxins, like *parabens* (found in personal care products) and *phthalates* (found in various plastics), have a complex nature in terms of their solubility. Mercury, for example, a risk associated with the consumption of fish and seafood, can be water- and fat-soluble, depending on its form. Inorganic mercury salts are water-soluble and cause intestinal (gut) irritation and severe kidney damage. Organic mercury compounds are fat-soluble and can cross the blood-brain barrier, causing neurological damage.[1] Regardless of the toxin, increased toxicity puts an immense strain on our organs, especially the liver, and is a huge risk factor for many conditions, including weight gain and diabetes.[2] Additionally, being overweight provides an easy reservoir for toxins to accumulate in our bodies. Some of these toxins directly interfere with our hormones and others with our neurological processes, impacting our moods, emotions, and even behavior. In all cases, food can provide a primary gateway for both reducing the incoming toxicity and optimizing the regular removal of toxins.

Like everything else in life, the body thrives when things are in balance; in the body, this is called *homeostasis*. In every moment, the body works to maintain or bring back its own biochemical balanced state. When we support our bodies with proper dietary and lifestyle habits, this process is easily maintained and normally equates to good physical, mental, and emotional health. When physical, mental, and emotional stressors exceed the body's coping ability, things begin to malfunction. The body may have to perpetually try to catch up, depleting its various resources; over time, this results in disease. The most common biochemical imbalances include the hormones and our neurotransmitters, as mentioned above, and the acid-alkaline balance, which we will cover in Chapter 4. In our society, female hormonal health has, perhaps, been the most distinct indicator of the negative impacts of poor food and lifestyle choices. It begins with the premature onset of puberty for many girls, spans the reproductive years with all sorts of menstrual cycle and fertility challenges, and often ends with a turbulent menopause. Thyroid hormone imbalances are another area of concern, leading to increased thyroid disease, especially amongst women. Our mental and emotional health balance also suffers, as some food ingredients and additives have neurotoxic, mood-altering, or hyperactive effects.

Excess weight or frequent or extreme weight fluctuations put stress and strain on the body, including all organs and tissues. When weight goes up or down, the body must adapt, taxing the cardiovascular, endocrine, respiratory, and digestive systems. Excess weight is most commonly attributed to consuming an excessive amount of calories, specifically nutrient-deficient ones, but it can also be caused by other stressors like the toxicity discussed above. Either way, once this becomes a concern for us, it can easily influence and give rise to other states of imbalance, resulting in disease.

By now, you have no doubt concluded that we rarely experience one of the five diet-related problems in isolation. There is usually a cascading effect: One problem, disease, or condition influences the formation of another. This is why paying serious and conscious attention to food choices is so vital today. It can be one of the most influential aspects of our health. With every food and drink you ingest, you are either supporting your body—reducing inflammation, oxidative stress, toxicity, and imbalances—or harming your body by increasing these. Every day, you have the choice to provide your body with a healing and preventative environment by making healthy eating a priority. The question now is: What does healthy eating mean?

The Confusion of Healthy

Accompanying the confusion that has been created by various groups, individuals, and the media, another factor contributes to the problem of contradictory information when it comes to healthy eating: the actual definition of *healthy*. What many of us may not realize is that while everyone seems to use this word, it, in no way, represents the same idea across all boards. For example, "healthy" lost some serious credibility when fast food restaurants began using it indiscriminately to highlight their menu items. How it is used by a medical doctor versus a naturopathic doctor; between a pharmacist versus an acupuncturist; between you versus your friend shows even more disparity, and it is not at all necessarily equivalent in its meaning. We each have our own unique perspective when it comes to healthiness, depending on numerous variables. In its simplicity, we know it refers to something that is good for us, but what we consider "good for us" opens up an even bigger can of worms. Therefore, when we hear someone say, "healthy," we cannot automatically assume it will fit our personal needs or standards. There is no one, clear, universal definition of the word.

For the most part, the definition used by doctors, organizations, and most individuals is based on presently accepted, common societal norms. From this perspective, the general concept of healthiness applies when one eats according to the four food groups: grains, fruits and vegetables, dairy, and meat and alternatives. Anything outside these groups is considered a treat or acceptable in moderation. As we get more specific, though, we begin to encounter a variety of subtle and gross differences as to the specific foods that are considered healthy in each of these groups, as well as their quality and mode of preparation. Each party brings into this equation their personal conditioning based on education, family upbringing, societal influence, and/or cultural tradition.

Many also define healthy food as that which their parents or grandparents ate. Inaccurate conclusions are often drawn based on this way of thinking, as so much has changed in even just the last few decades. Not only has science and research advanced to shed new light on how our bodies interact with food, but the quality of our food has diminished tremendously. We must consider today the effects of modern farming and food-processing methods, toxicity, as well as current sustainability issues. Your parents or grandparents may have consumed milk and meat, but today's milk and meat are not the same your ancestors drank and ate, nor are the quantities consumed of each, while living so sedentarily. Today's fruits and vegetables are not grown in the same clean, fertile, mineral-rich soils, without the use of synthetic fertilizers and pesticides. Today, we are presented with an unprecedented amount of processed food, teeming with added sugar and salt. For these reasons alone, we cannot base our definition of healthy on what our recent ancestors ate.

Others go even further and define healthy as what the earliest humans ate, but the truth is that the further we go, the less we know for certain what people ate, how much they ate, and the general state of their health and longevity. There are some smart fundamentals we should consider from the past, but they must be analyzed in light of our modern needs and challenges.

Again, I want to emphasize that, for the most part, the worst and most confusing usage of what healthy means has a lot to do with processed food items or those that carry a large financial stake, like animal products. The information passed around by science, medical, and governing experts goes around in circles, with the root influence coming from the corporations trying to sell whatever products they can. People argue about what is considered healthy based on their personal identities, stakes and gains. For one example, we can consider butter and margarine. The industry sends us dancing in circles, trying to figure out which one is the healthy choice. The same problem does not exist for, say, broccoli and cabbage or apples and oranges. The latter examples are healthy at their most inherent level, and no fad or industry bias is going to change that. Let's take a closer look at butter versus margarine.

Modern margarine is typically comprised of refined oils, which commonly include genetically modified ingredients. It doesn't matter how many healthy omega-3 fats, vitamins, or probiotics they add to it or that it has zero cholesterol or trans fat; all that is simply used to distract us from the foundation of what this product really is: a highly refined and problematic food, not to mention entirely unnecessary. The following is an ingredient list from a popular margarine company:

> Canola and sunflower oils 74 percent, water, modified palm and palm kernel oils 6 percent, salt 1.8 percent, whey protein concentrate 1.4 percent, soy lecithin 0.2 percent, vegetable monoglycerides, potassium sorbate, vegetable color, artificial flavor, citric acid, Vitamin A palmitate, Vitamin D3, alpha-tocopherol acetate (Vitamin E).

Oils, in and of themselves, are processed food products, regardless of how healthy they are, as we will explore in Chapter 14. This product further processes them, creating a chemically fabricated final product that is inflammatory in nature. In no way can this be deemed healthy, at least not if we are serious about healing and prevention.

Butter, on the other hand, has been made and consumed for centuries, albeit in smaller quantities than what is eaten and used today. Those who see it as a natural dairy food classify it as healthy. Those who see it as an animal-derived saturated fat classify it as unhealthy. Regardless of which perspective you prefer, today's conventional butter comes from factory-farmed cows that have been fed pesticides and/or genetically modified ingredients, as well as given various drugs and hormones. The extracted product then undergoes a heavy processing, pasteurization, and chemical alteration. To top it off, we consume a great abundance of butter today, too regularly. If, on the other hand, you source out raw butter from local, organic cows, that is a different story. This is not the norm, however, for the majority of butter consumers, so we cannot apply the term healthy to butter either.

The point I am trying to make is that each of us can come to similar conclusions and know what to put into our bodies and what not to if we are only willing to consciously look at the food we eat with some discernment. Whether it is common sense, logic, or intuition, I really believe each of us has the ability to reason out what healthy most accurately represents. Reasoning this way and applying some critical thinking skills can be greatly empowering, as long as we choose to use these tools wisely.

Finally, healthy can also refer to various states of being, depending on the person. Some still consider themselves healthy if they get only a few colds a year or if they cannot sleep properly or make it through the day without stimulants. Others think they are healthy because they are only on one medication, while their friend is on four. Some feel healthy just because they have not been diagnosed with a disease, in spite of frequent emotional outbursts and an inability to maintain relationships. Not only have we forgotten what healthy food is, but we have also forgotten what it actually means to be a healthy human being. This does not mean that we are aiming for some static state of perfection, but simply that we can do so much better. Our range and frequency of acute and chronic physical, mental, and emotional conditions is overwhelming. Something is definitely missing in our definition of healthy.

What Happened to Healthy?

As mentioned above, healthy can mean many different things to different people. In my opinion, the term has lost much of its worth, credibility, and meaning. It is tossed around without most of us realizing what it truly means in relation to the body and the mind. This normally happens because we are inundated unconsciously by various media messages and societal conditioning that provides us with an onslaught of various illusions of healthiness. Let me give you another example of the problem.

In teaching about nutrition, whether to groups or one on one, I often hear about some person someone knew that seemed to eat healthy yet still develop some sort of debilitating disease, building the case that healthy eating doesn't really work. We all seem to have this particular example in our lives, leading us to believe that healthy eating may be overrated or just not worth it. But let's peel back a few layers. As you noticed, the subtitle of this book contains the word "holistic." Holistic health includes the influence of the mind and spirit, as well as the body, but it also includes the social and environmental aspects. In regard to health, this means we are applying a broader analysis, which includes the numerous multifactorial layers that impact us daily, as well as their interconnected nature. Even though my journey into health and nutrition did not start with the holistic perspective, today I cannot imagine it without the inclusion of this crucial element. Once we see our multidimensional nature, we can begin to appreciate and understand the often unexplainable occurrences, like a healthy-eating person still being afflicted with disease. Now, let's go back to that famous example of ours.

When you observe and label how someone eats, bear in mind that you are gauging it based on your own filters, your own definition of healthy, as you see it. If you are told by another that they eat healthy, you must rely on what that means to them. Unfortunately, most people are not fully aware of what, how much, or how poorly they actually eat on a daily basis, providing an unreliable source of data to begin with. We are busy and stressed, and our vision of our eating habits is often a much more digestible version for us rather than the reality, no pun intended. When asked to keep track of their food intake for several days, many are shocked to find just how out of balance they are eating. The point is that there is a lot you do not know about another person and their lifestyle and eating habits, even if you live with them, particularly because we, ourselves, are not always able to be objective. For the most accurate understanding of why a person may get a disease, we must consider the afflicted's way of life, stress levels, exercise levels, chemical exposure, emotional patterns, childhood traumas, and, most importantly, thought patterns in both the conscious and subconscious mind before we make any concluding judgments. When we assess someone's life or health on the basis of surface-level observations or passing comments, it presents us with a very flawed version of reality.

We are simply working with an incomplete picture when we observe people who seem to eat poorly yet appear perfectly healthy or ones who seem to eat healthy yet suffer from one or more conditions. Unless we study and understand each person on a proper holistic level, we are not in a very good position to draw conclusions. It is neither good science nor good logic to rely on surface-level observations as the basis for our findings, assumptions, and determinations. We are each unique in regard to our lifestyle choices, and all of us are differently affected by our environment. So, while generalizations can help us make sense of things, they can also be very harmful, misleading us to build false correlations.

When it comes to food, there is no doubt that it plays a major role in shaping our health and longevity. However, there are other factors involved, like the quantity and quality of our sleep, exercise, stress, chemical exposure, and thinking or mind patterns—the basis of the complete, holistic foundation. Many are quick to blame genetics when they are prone to or seem unable to overcome a weight condition or disease. This, too, requires a more in-depth look.

Thanks to the field of *epigenetics*, we know today that genes are primarily influenced by their environment. The food you eat, the thoughts you have, and the chemicals to which you expose yourself all play a part in turning genetic factors on and off, and this can result in better or worse health for you. The most prominent reason why certain conditions run in families, according to what we've learned thus far, is that families share common habits, from the way we eat to the way we think. It is very empowering to know that we are in no way slaves to our genes or our external environment. We simply need to take responsibility for the choices we make and strive to connect the dots as to the consequences of each of our actions.

In this book, I will provide you with a foundation for healthy eating. This, alone, has the potential to make a huge difference in the quality of your life when it comes to your health and wellbeing. In Part 3, we will address other factors beyond food, so you will walk away with a more complete understanding of how to heal and prevent disease and support optimal weight and wellness. For optimal health, all areas—physical, emotional, mental, and spiritual—require and deserve proper attention and balance.

So What Does Health Really Mean?

As we continue to delve deeper, we must understand what *health* means, optimal health, to be more specific. For the majority of people, health is simply the absence of disease or any of its obvious physical symptoms; however, the true definition is much broader than that. As of 1948, the World Health Organization (WHO) has defined health as "a state of complete physical, mental, and social wellbeing and not merely the absence of disease or infirmity." This is the foundation of a wonderful explanation that has often been forgotten today. Expanding on this broader definition, health is also the abundance of energy and vitality; emotional wellbeing; graceful aging; and physical agility. Being optimally healthy means having an effective immune system that can protect you properly, so that you will not be victimized by infectious disease cycles or cause you to live in fear of your natural environment. It means having a digestive system that can efficiently digest, assimilate, and eliminate. It means having clarity of mind, a good memory, and sharp focus and concentration. It means not having to rely on chemical or synthetic substances to keep your body functioning properly. It means not needing regular stimulants to improve your energy levels or mood. When we learn to see health in this fuller context, we begin to see, even more clearly, how our modern eating and lifestyle habits are simply not working toward achieving this broader version of health.

When it comes to the definition of healthy as it applies to food, a similar approach needs to be taken, to offer a holistic and complete view. My definition of healthy eating, the way I see it and how I will refer to it throughout this book, will be explained below. It is the most thorough definition I have arrived at to this point, after an extensive examination of data, research, and personal experience. This definition takes into consideration the body's needs, as well as our modern food and social challenges.

When it comes to food, healthy means:

• Food that is nutrient-rich, as opposed to calorie-rich.

• Food that is wholesome, natural, and pure.

- Food that *is* the ingredient or is made up solely of ingredients that are wholesome, natural, and pure.

- Food that is not chemically or genetically altered in any way that compromises its nutritional integrity or safety.

- Food that is most in alignment with our bodies' anatomy and physiology.

- Food that is most in alignment with our personal evolution and planetary sustainability.

Learning How to Eat Healthy

On our journey toward optimal health, we will integrate the above points that address what healthy food should look like in practical terms. If you treat my definition like a checklist, you will know you are on an optimally healthy track if you can check off each point for your food of interest. Once you know what healthy food should consist of, you can engage in truly healthy eating. You will nourish your body with healthy food from a wide variety of healthy sources daily.

This book is divided into three parts, each of which provides explanations for all the information and choices presented. In Part 1, we will cover how we should eat to heal, prevent disease, and maintain optimal health and weight. In Part 2, we will narrow our focus and get more specific, learning what to eat. Finally, in Part 3, we will expand our focus to include and embrace other holistic factors, lifestyle habits, and practical life tips for making it all work.

Here is a summary of Part 1 – How to Eat:

1. **Eat Natural**
2. **Eat Plant-Based**
3. **Eat Acid-Alkaline Balanced**
4. **Eat Raw**
5. **Eat Organic**

We will explore each point over the course of the next five chapters. As we come to understand each of the five ways of eating, you will learn how to make the right choices for yourself, and what constitutes an optimal approach to eating. We will simplify and clarify the foundation of nutrition so you can be empowered and confident that healthy eating can be easy, logical, and possible for all. We simply need to peel back all the layers of unnecessary information, misinformation, conditioning, and diet fads to take back our natural response of knowing how to feed ourselves for healing, prevention, and optimal wellbeing.

CHAPTER 2
Eating Natural

Eating natural means eating real, whole food, and it is the polar opposite of eating processed. To some extent, we all know that processed or heavily refined food is not healthy for us and that we should minimize or avoid it. In other words, I am not going to tell you anything new here. However, even though we may have heard this and know it, we do not necessarily apply it in our everyday diets. We may respond with a glazed-over, "I know, I know," but how many of us are showing in our daily eating habits that we really do know? Oftentimes, a nod, a yawn, and simple agreement is about as far as this knowing goes. Some people get defensive, others offer excuses for their choices, and still others just feel helpless to turn things around. Regardless, too many of us are using processed food as our main food source on a regular basis. One reason we do not take this message more seriously is that many of us are not fully aware of what actually constitutes processed food, especially since it has become so prevalent. Another reason is that we may not fully realize how processed food really destroys our health and why it is completely inferior to wholesome, natural food.

People in most modern, developed countries depend on health and government agencies to regulate which substances are safe for internal human consumption or external exposure and which aren't. In North America, we have governing bodies like the FDA, USDA, and Health Canada to guide us and supposedly keep us safe from harmful substances, or at least this is what most would like to believe. Consequently, most of us think that if processed food or its various ingredients were that bad, surely our governments and health agencies would not allow them to be sold or recommended. Or would they?

This is where there is a huge and detrimental disconnect in our system. Governments complain about rising healthcare costs, yet they do little to tackle healthy eating and preventative care at the root level. Instead, they attempt to implement health solutions that often waste more money and resources than any value they offer. Part of this problem is that there are simply too many corporate connections in politics today. Real change does not happen simply because it would be bad for business. There are strong, binding ties between governments, corporations, and regulating agencies, all of which have their own priorities and interests to protect. This is why every one of us must be accountable for our choices and take responsibility for our own health; even though most of the processed food out there has no business being on our store shelves, it is, because it is somebody's business. Without delving any deeper into the political and corporate side of things, we simply need to understand that the system is far from perfect, and it is up to each one of us to make the right decisions for ourselves. Every choice we make from now on will shape the system. Many people complain, waiting for the system to get better, but if we become overweight or develop a disease and decrease our quality of life, there is no use in blaming the external for the choices we have made and the consequences we have to live with. The more conscious and aware we become about how and why things work as they do, the better we can make intelligent choices that will result in desirable consequences, rather than just accepting outdated or biased information as the truth and making ignorant choices based upon it. As leading nutrition researcher T. Colin Campbell, PhD shares in the book he co-wrote with health educator Howard Jacobson, PhD, *Whole: Rethinking the Science of Nutrition*, "the crucial shift in the way we think about our health will happen one person at a time."

A Case of Nutrients

The biggest problem when it comes to processed foods is that they are *nutrient deficient*. This means the vital nutrients your body most depends on for healing and prevention—like natural vitamins, minerals, phytonutrients, and antioxidants—are minimally present at best or absent altogether. Many of these nutrients are sensitive to heat, oxidation, and other factors; thus, they are easily lost or destroyed during food-processing procedures. Some are simply not present to begin with, due to the low quality of the original ingredients or their heavily refined nature. Even macronutrients, like fats and carbohydrates, are inferior in processed foods, as they often come in the form of refined fats and sugars. That would be bad enough on its own, but to add to this, most of these foods are very high in calories as well. As we will discuss in Chapter 17, not all calories are created equal, and those found in processed food are the worst, as they are highly nutrient deficient and, thus, provide far more energy than nutrients. The lack of nutrients keeps our body nutritionally unsatisfied, which can easily result in overeating. This is blatantly obvious in our rampant health and weight problems. As the now-famous saying goes, "we are overfed but undernourished." To add even more fuel to the fire, most processed foods, if not all of them, are *highly inflammatory*.

To explain this idea, let's use the example of boxed cereals. Most people in our society eat them on a daily basis and feed these refined cereals to their children from an early age. Looking at the nutrition label, you will typically read that the product is low in fat, made with whole grains, and has some fiber, protein, vitamins, and minerals. What could be wrong with that? It sounds like it provides everything you need, right? Based on the nutrition facts label and package claims, the product does not seem so bad at all. In fact, it wins most of us over with how healthy it appears to be.

It isn't until one looks at the ingredient list that the story takes on more clarity. You will discover that most of the vitamins and minerals in the product did not come from the actual food; rather, they have been added in as isolated, synthetic compounds. The product has at least one added sugar, though there are typically multiple sugars added. There are modified food ingredients, ingredients we cannot pronounce or understand, colors, flavors, and preservatives. Even though almost all boxed cereals today claim they are "whole grain," what they contain is a very poor representation of what whole grains are. When we look inside the boxes of popular choices, we see something that resembles pet food pellets of various shapes, sizes, and even colors; processed grain products with no visible whole grains at all. Perhaps the product did once come from a whole grain, but the product sitting in your breakfast cupboard is a far cry from that. We are not even taking into consideration how the original ingredients were grown, their level of quality, or the processing they had to undergo. While this may not sound like a big deal to you, it is a very big deal to your body in terms of how your cells will recognize, digest, and assimilate this food item.

Other processed food examples are not as drastic, though many are much more so. If we pick up a frozen food entrée that includes some mashed potatoes, beef slices, and vegetables, we may be hard pressed to see the problem; it all seems like real food. The nutrition label may sound just fine too. Again, the story takes a different turn when we examine the ingredients, revealing that the supposed three-ingredient meal is actually composed of far more than the pretty picture on the box. These additional ingredients typically include various additives, modified food ingredients, genetically modified ingredients, refined oils, sugars, and salt. You are given no information about the quality of the original ingredients or how they were stored, handled, cooked or processed for you. Due to the nature of processing, companies can afford to source the cheapest ingredients and hide many flaws that would not be so easily disguised if you were looking at the ingredients in the produce or fresh meat section of your store.

We really don't need to get into the more drastic examples. Whether it is a canned soup, common bread, salad dressing, boxed cereal, or frozen meal, the lesson is very simple: Look at your food, and if your food comes with an ingredient label, examine and read it carefully. If the food does not look wholesome and natural and/or the ingredients do not sound wholesome and natural, allow your innate knowing to kick in, recognizing that it does not belong in your body! Going to the root of all food in such a way will help us make smart choices. Aside from using a process of logical inquiry and observation to examine your food item, the ingredient list is where you will learn the most about your food in a meaningful way. Although the required nutrition facts label can provide some guidance, overall, it has proven to cause more harm than good. As we will learn in Chapter 17, it is often a major source of confusion and misleading information about our food.

A Case of Chemicals

We have come to prioritize and so heavily rely on convenience within the food sector that we often do not realize how much it is hurting us, defeating its role as a helpful innovation to begin with. When it comes to processed foods, they are only good-looking, great-tasting, and long-lasting thanks to a mixture of chemicals and synthetic compounds. It only takes one glance at the ingredient list of nearly any processed food item to prove this; in most cases, the more processed the food is, the more chemical names you will find.

As we try to read and decipher these foreign chemical names, we may squirm or get a little uncomfortable. Ultimately, however, we often feel they must be safe, or else our governing agencies would not allow them to be included in our food. If you recall, as I shared at the start of this chapter, we have quite the interesting system when it comes to health, food safety, and regulation. Without using this book to dissect its strengths and weaknesses, let's get proactive instead and simply understand that the governing agencies have their own priorities and agendas, just as you have yours. Unfortunately, these priorities often fail to align with the consumer's optimal health. In the end, though, no one is responsible for your choices but you. You must be 100 percent accountable for yourself and your health! This requires that you think for yourself, rather than letting others do the thinking for you. It will take some effort and initiative at first as you learn to make smart choices for your optimal wellbeing, but I assure you that it will quickly become second nature to you.

Various chemicals are used in processed foods, and these can lead to increased toxicity in our bodies. Some of these are safe, some are assumed safe, and some are blatantly unsafe. As a group, they are commonly called "additives," and they are added to our food for one or more of the following reasons:

1. **To maintain product consistency or texture.** (Example: emulsifiers or anti-caking agents)

2. **To improve nutritional value.** (Example: synthetic vitamins)

3. **To prevent spoilage and maintain palatability.** (Example: preservatives)

4. **To provide leavening or control the acidity levels.** (Example: rising agents)

5. **To enhance or bring out a flavor.** (Example: natural or artificial flavors)

6. **To provide a desired look.** (Example: artificial colors or glazing agents)

While all of these may sound like viable, justifiable reasons for adding these substances, why can't we just enjoy the natural taste, texture, and look of the food? The truth is that we are greatly disconnected from our food as a society;

we demand that our juices be brighter, our breads fluffier, our sauces thicker. It may behoove us, though, to imagine what the food looks like after processing, before the finishing touches. When food is heavily processed, it very quickly loses its original appeal. Have you ever tried to blend one too many fruits together or cooked something a bit too long? Personal experience quickly indicates that our food loses its natural look, taste, texture, and nutritional value when it is over-treated. Now, imagine what happens to food when it is processed on a large scale. If we saw and tasted those processed foods without any of the pretty colors, flavors, and texture agents they add, most of us would want nothing to do with it.

Even if we could do without the colors, flavors, and texture agents that give the food its general appeal, the same does not easily hold true for food preservatives. Many argue that it is impossible to fulfill the needs of our large and ever-growing human population without the use of preservatives. However, this can be avoided or drastically reduced as well, if we are only willing to take more responsibility for our food. Otherwise, we will continue to pay the price of convenience with the most prized currency we have: our health.

Real, natural food comes from living materials; naturally, these deteriorate and break down within a short period of time. This is Mother Nature's clue for us as to when it is best to eat the food for maximum health and nutritional benefits. In our corporately driven world today, the number-one goal of making and selling any product is primarily profit. If a product must be transported long distance, then sit on a shelf for an extended period of time, it has a high potential of spoiling, resulting in profit loss. The other side of this coin is that people today also expect and demand a certain level of unrealistic convenience. When we buy a food product, we want it to last an unnatural amount of time, as we have no desire for our busy lives to be inconvenienced by the natural breakdown process. We enable this cycle with our demands and are often part of the problem, along with the processed food companies.

All this focus on preservation has provided us with food that is so well preserved that it has a hard time breaking down within a healthy or normal period of time. While some may declare this as an amazing scientific accomplishment, we must consider what these substances are doing within our bodies. While theoretically most food preservatives are generally recognized as safe, our health and many studies have told us otherwise. For example, nitrates/ nitrites alone (preservatives common in processed meats like cold cuts and sausages) have been found, on numerous occasions, to be directly linked with health problems. A study conducted in 2009 and published in the *Journal of Alzheimer's Disease* found a direct link between nitrates and increased deaths from diseases like Alzheimer's, Type 2 diabetes, and Parkinson's.[1] Other studies have linked these preservatives to various cancers.[2] These questionable preservatives are also one of the reasons why popular health organizations like the American Cancer Society and Physicians Committee for Responsible Medicine advise against the consumption of processed meats. While I could share with you study after study about this or that preservative, it is safe to say that natural food is the innate, easy, and logical choice. We should not have to be convinced with data and studies that it has a much higher value than anything that comes off of an assembly line in a box, can, or package.

We simply need to take back our food and go back to a more natural way of eating. It does not take a genius to figure out that foods based on foreign substances will not lead to healthy outcomes, despite what anyone says about their safety. We need to respect food's natural look, taste, and shelf life and demand more natural food. After all, how far are we going to allow the processed food to go? We are already aware of genetic manipulation within the food supply, pushing the boundaries of our food production in ever more dangerous directions. Something has to give, or else we run the risk of causing permanent damage to the food supply, not to mention our potential to survive on this planet.

When it comes to processed food, commit to releasing excuses that aim to justify consuming substances that simply do not belong in the body or aid the body in working optimally. Most of these substances are the leading contributors of our inflammation, oxidative stress, increased toxicity, weight gain, and various imbalances and diseases over time.

A Case of Sodium

Another major factor that should deter us from consuming a diet based on processed food is the high sodium level. Sodium is widely used in processed food, and this goes back to our previous section on food additives. Sodium and its many derivatives, like sodium chloride or monosodium glutamate, are additives used to achieve two outcomes: preserve the food and enhance the flavor. It is almost impossible to pick up a processed food item today and not see some salt or sodium listed in the ingredients. It is also next to impossible to examine a nutrition facts label and find the sodium level to be lower than the number of calories per serving. Why is this important? Allow me to explain.

When it comes to sodium, while experts are still divided as to the exact value that defines a healthy sodium intake, most agree that it should be no more than 2,000 mg of sodium daily. Such a value is more than sufficient to fulfill our minimum sodium requirement without causing excessive harm. The American Heart Association (AHA) goes even further, recommending no more than 1,500 mg of sodium per day in order to reduce the risk of cardiovascular disease and high blood pressure.[3] The AHA also shares that the current average sodium consumption in the United States is around 3,400 mg a day, more than double the recommended value.

When we become aware of the drastic amount of sodium used in processed food, the excess of sodium in the modern diet is obvious. Nutrition facts labels present numbers based on the assumption that the average adult consumes 2,000 calories per day. Naturally, many people eat more than this, and some eat less, but this does not change the point. Think about what this means when one's diet consists primarily of processed foods. The sodium in most processed foods is at least 1.5 to 2 (or more) times higher than the number of calories. (Check out the average pasta sauce if you want a real shocker.) Therefore, if you eat 2,000 calories of processed food daily, you are consuming an average 4,000 mg of sodium every 24 hours! Excess sodium disrupts our sodium-potassium balance, which is responsible for many cell reactions. It has been linked to increased hypertension (high blood pressure) and heart disease, muscle and bone loss, and consequential osteoporosis. According to Dr. Joel Fuhrman, medical nutrition expert and author of *Eat to Live*, salt may increase the inflammation associated with several autoimmune conditions.[4]

The sodium overabundance applies to every processed food, from bread to ice cream and everything in between. No matter where we look, when it comes to processed food, the sodium levels are grossly excessive. On top of the processed food consumed, a large portion of our sodium intake also comes from the foods consumed in restaurants, including any prepared food or takeout. You can inquire about your meal choices to learn about their sodium levels, but many restaurants still do not have the capability to provide accurate and thorough nutrition data. There has been an attempt by some governing bodies in North America to enforce a mandatory reduction of sodium in products. This is a great step in the right direction, but it is not something we can afford to rely on or wait for. Take accountability for your personal choices and, in turn, your health.

But how can you be accountable? What can you do? Besides drastically reducing or completely eliminating processed foods from your diet, if you do pick up any packaged food with a nutrition facts label, check the calorie-to-sodium ratio. The general rule of thumb is as follows:

> The sodium amount should be less than—or, at worst, equal to—the number of calories per serving.

You are thinking of a 1:1 sodium-to-calorie ratio, with the goal being a sodium number that is much lower than the calorie number. For example, if a slice of bread is 120 calories, you want the sodium amount to be less than 120 mg. There is one main scenario to be mindful of when applying this rule. You must take into consideration the total sodium amount per serving. If you eat four slices of this bread, you will consume roughly one-quarter to one-third of your daily sodium allowance, and we are not even taking into account what that bread is eaten with or what the rest of your day's food will consist of. Likewise, a food item with 600 calories and 500 mg of sodium per serving fits the general rule of thumb, but that sodium amount already accounts for about one-third of your sodium intake for the day, making it a very high-sodium food; also, if that item does not comprise your whole meal, it may be too high in calories as well. Other than that, if your diet is almost solely composed of whole, natural foods and you decide to have one processed food item that day that fails to conform to the sodium rule above, it should not be a problem, provided that the bulk of your daily diet comes from non-processed, whole, natural, homemade meals, where the salt shaker is used very sparingly, if at all.

Of course, it is not natural to check or count sodium-to-calorie amounts, and it can make eating a tedious event. (We'll explore the numbers game in Chapter 17.) One of the best things about choosing a natural food diet is that it provides us with a naturally low sodium diet, with no sodium to check or count.

Natural Food Is the Natural Way to Go

We cannot forget that our bodies (organs, tissues, and cells) recognize food compounds most easily and can use them most effectively in their most natural state. We started out on this planet as living beings, consuming living things, and we have evolved from there. In just the last seventy-five years or so, our bodies have been subjected to highly processed, foreign, and unnatural food. Perhaps over the next few thousand years, humans will evolve to eat chemically enhanced, genetically modified, nutrient-depleted food and maintain their health. Personally, though, I don't think the human body will ever live to see such a day. We have to go back to Mother Nature and our own nature, to go back to eating what is best suited for our bodies and our health. This doesn't mean negating the progress we have made or trying to re-create the diets of our ancient ancestors. Rather, it means taking the best of ancient practices along with modern wisdom and evolution of the human being and combining it with the most sustainable approach for our planet. If you want fruits and vegetables, eat *real* fruits and vegetables rather than fruit-flavored bars, frozen vegetable pies, or gummy fruit snacks. If you want grains, eat *real* grains, not processed breads, crackers, or boxed cereals.

Our bodies know what they are doing when it comes to keeping us healthy, but for them to do so, we must give them the right support and tools to work with. Just think of what would happen if you tried to build a house with inferior materials, perhaps rotting wood or porous bricks. While you might be able to throw the house together, it will not be structurally sound, and you will be faced with serious problems, frequent renovations, or the risk of complete collapse. With every meal, you are building the quality of your body and, thus, your health. Make them count in your favor!

Practical Tips for Eating Natural

To finish this section, here are some practical tips for making the best choices when it comes to choosing the most natural, wholesome foods:

1. **Read all your ingredient labels.** All ingredients should be just as real as the intended food item. The more additives, chemicals, preservatives, and unknown and long words you see on the label, the more that food should be avoided.

2. **Shop in the whole food sections of the grocery store.** In the past, a general health tip was to shop on the periphery of the grocery store, since most whole, natural foods tend to be located there. This includes fruits, vegetables, bulk seeds and nuts, etc. The inner aisles are full of boxes, cans, and packages that make up what we refer to as processed food. However, there are some major exceptions to this rule, and that can make things a bit more difficult. Processed meat, dairy, various frozen foods, and most breads are on the periphery, while dry, whole grains and beans, herbs, and spices are in the inner aisles. This is why it is important to learn where whole, natural foods are located in your favorite grocery store and stick solely to those areas.

3. **Choose foods that are in, or as close as possible to, their natural state.** If you want potatoes, choose fresh potatoes and cook them at home in a healthy way. Avoid French fries, frozen potato-based meals, seasoned, or powdered potatoes or canned potato soup. Other examples include apples rather than apple cakes or apple juice; steel-cut oats instead of instant oatmeal or boxed cereals; dry beans and grains instead of canned or precooked ones; raw nuts and seeds instead of roasted and seasoned options, etc.

4. **Eat fresh as much as possible.** Fresh food has the highest nutrient density, with the highest amount of its natural nutrients present and active. The more processed a food is, the fewer original nutrients it will contain. Some are so nutrient depleted that they have to be fortified with synthetic nutrients. Choose fresh fruits and vegetables over frozen, canned, or

precooked. Unprocessed, whole frozen are the second-best choice, but avoid the other options completely. If you choose to eat fish, pick fresh over canned or processed. Whatever the food may be, focus on choosing the most natural, wholesome, fresh form possible.

5. **Shop in the natural sections of the grocery store.** An increasing number of grocery stores are beginning to include a natural foods section. These areas contain convenience foods that fall into this category, such as whole, organic, non-GMO, gluten-free, and preservative-free options. While they may still include many processed foods, they are normally much better choices than their conventional counterparts and can serve as great transition items for someone who is switching from a processed to a natural food diet. There are also many natural health food stores that offer some great quality, wholesome, natural food options. However, don't be too easily influenced by the new wave of fancy health claims within this marketplace. Processed food is processed food, regardless of its source or allure.

Apply these tips to make smart choices and be a wise, discerning consumer. Allow your food to nourish you, heal you, and protect you from inflammation, invading organisms, environmental damage, and breakdown. Remember that we are making an impact with our choices every day, shaping the current and future landscape of the system that will be available to us. For all these reasons and more, natural food is the natural way to go.

CHAPTER 3
Eating Plant-Based

Eating plant-based means the majority of your food comes from plants. Plant-based can include vegetarian and vegan lifestyles, though this is not always the case. How you choose to approach a plant-based diet and which animal foods, if any, you choose to include or exclude will be a very personal choice. Whether you choose to go 100 percent plant-based (vegan) will depend on your personal decisions, needs, and values. For the time being, listen to your body and your inner guidance with respect to where you need to be right now. Remember that this is a journey. As our level of awareness grows, as our lives change, and as our society continues to transform, we may find that new paths begin to make the most sense to us, paths we never would have planned to take. That is the power of growth, change, and evolution.

In mainstream thinking, the notion and value of plant-based was initially commonly associated with The Mediterranean Diet, which emphasizes eating primarily plant-based foods, such as fruits and vegetables, whole grains, legumes, and nuts. However, leading-edge, nutrition-oriented physicians, nutritionists, and alternative health experts have been promoting plant-based eating for decades. Drs. Dean Ornish, Joel Fuhrman, Gabriel Cousens, Caldwell Esselstyn, and T. Colin Campbell are among these leaders, and some of these names may ring familiar. These forerunners dedicated their lives and work to educating the public about the power of whole-food, plant-based eating for maintaining optimal health and preventing and reversing disease. In 2011, with the release of *Forks Over Knives*, a documentary directed by Lee Fulkerson, plant-based eating was given a serious boost. If you have not yet seen the film, I highly recommend it. Nutrition science has always known the high value of plant foods, especially fruits and vegetables, but we are just now beginning to grasp the full scope of why this is so. As health in our society and the health of our planet faces some of its greatest challenges yet, it has never been more vital than now to shift our attention to a plant-based way of eating.

Why Plant-Based?

Plants have been used as both food and medicine since humans began their journey on this planet. We most likely know that fruits and vegetables are really good for us, but we probably are not aware of why or just how good. Not only are they great-tasting and satisfying, but they are nature's greatest gift to us when it comes to nourishment, healing, and prevention. The science of nutrition continues to discover and learn about their unique characteristics to this day; it is likely we have only skimmed the surface of their yet-to-be-discovered full potential. All whole plant foods are powerhouses full of vital nutrients, particularly vitamins, minerals, antioxidants, and phytonutrients. When it comes to nutrient density, they easily trump animal-derived and processed foods. While their nutrient levels are very high, calories tend to be very low, making them ideal foods for the maintenance of optimal weight and health.

In terms of vitamins and minerals, all plants foods have richly unique profiles of micronutrients. Fruits, vegetables, herbs, and spices tend to be the dominant sources of Vitamins A, C, E, K, and folate, but most of them contain some amounts of nearly every vitamin and mineral. Nuts, seeds, beans, legumes, and grains tend to be dominant sources of minerals and B vitamins. Therefore, it is not helpful for us to get attached to specific foods as specific sources of micronutrients, like oranges being a source of Vitamin C or almonds being a source of calcium. This narrow view completely undermines their potential as each plant food is a source of most of them. Really, the only two limited micronutrients seem to be Vitamin D, whose primary source for us is the sun, and Vitamin B12, whose primary source are certain bacteria.

Plants contain *phytonutrients*, also called *phytochemicals*—nutrient compounds that are unique to them. Phytonutrients are not vitamins or minerals; rather, they are a unique category of nutrients. They are a relatively new concept for most people, as science continues its own exploration and understanding of them. It is estimated that there are thousands of phytonutrients, and we are continuously discovering new ones with remarkable benefits. Common phytonutrients include carotenoids, such as lutein and astaxanthin; flavonoids, resveratrol, coumarins, indoles, isoflavones, lignans, organosulfurs, and plant sterols.

Many of these have *antioxidant* properties, which is another reason why plant foods are so optimal for us; antioxidants are substances that protect the body from free radical damage. As we discussed in Chapter 1, oxidative stress caused by an excess of damaging free radicals is one of our greatest health threats. Some vitamins and minerals, like Vitamins A, C, E, and the mineral selenium also have antioxidant properties. The promise shown by phytonutrients and antioxidants thus far where our health, prevention, and disease reversal is concerned is astonishing! Some phytonutrients, like those found in the cruciferous family of vegetables, protect against cancers, even going so far as to prevent cancerous cells from multiplying. Others, like resveratrol, are linked with anti-aging and longevity benefits. Others are protective for the heart, immune system, and eyes. The more we learn about them, the more we will begin to fully understand why plant foods—whole, natural plant foods—are so good for every single area of our health. Not only should we eat a lot of them regularly, but we should eat them in their most nutritionally intact form; we cannot afford to destroy these amazing benefits with industrial processing.

As if all that isn't reason enough to base our diets on plant foods, all green plants have something else that is unique to them only: chlorophyll, life's natural elixir. As with our nutrient friends above, the power of this substance and its potential for us has not fully been tapped into, nor commonly understood. The molecular structure of chlorophyll is almost identical to that of hemoglobin in our blood. In 1915, Richard Willstätter won a Nobel Prize for showing that magnesium is held within the chlorophyll molecule in a very similar manner to the way iron is held in our blood hemoglobin. Further research indicated that chlorophyll actually helps rebuild and renew blood cells, possibly even proving valuable in cases of anemia. Although we do not know yet the full potential of this molecule, we do know that it has abundant benefits for our health, including antioxidant, anti-inflammatory, and wound-healing properties. On top of this, chlorophyll offers dozens of other beneficial functions, such as powerful detoxifying and cleansing; enhancing the immune system; working with vitamins and minerals in many beneficial reactions; and healing, growing, and promoting optimal functioning of cells, tissues, and organs. It is also highly alkalizing (a concept we will discuss in the next chapter) and energizing, improving feelings of overall wellbeing and vitality.

Finally, only plant foods (along with mushrooms, a fungi) contain fiber—a highly valuable component for our bodies. The tough, rigid part of plant cell walls is composed of a carbohydrate called *cellulose*, which we commonly refer to as fiber. It is not fully digestible for us, but that is part of what makes it so beneficial as it provides bulk within the intestines. Fiber is typically classified into two groups, soluble and insoluble, each of which has its own unique role in optimizing body functions. It supports our body's unique anatomy and physiology, specifically where our digestive tract is concerned, making fiber-rich plant foods highly protective against colon cancer. It enhances proper elimination, cleansing, detoxification, blood sugar levels, cholesterol levels, and weight maintenance. It helps us feel full faster and longer and positively supports healthy microflora communities in our intestines.

Our Evolutionary Plant-Based Journey

To date, a plant-based diet has been proven to be the most optimal, from a human health and planetary health perspective. Note, though, that this specifically refers to whole, natural plant foods, from fresh and living plant sources. As you can imagine, we can easily call a cereal-, bread-, and pasta-rich diet a plant-based diet, since these products are derived from plants, but this is not what most nutrition experts consider plant-based. An optimally healthy plant-based foundation is composed of vegetables. If you are just starting to explore the healing and preventative nature of plant-based eating, I highly recommend immersing yourself in more resources on this topic. While it is possible to hear something once and understand its value, repetition is normally necessary in order to experience a paradigm shift that propels us into effective action. You can follow up with resources from some of the plant-based expert names I mentioned at the start of this chapter. Some outstanding books that complement what I share in this book include *Eat to Live* by Dr. Joel Fuhrman, *Perfect Health: The Natural Way* by Mary-ann Shearer, *Whole: Rethinking the Science of Nutrition* by Dr. T. Colin Campbell, *Prevent and Reverse Heart Disease* by Dr. Caldwell B. Esselstyn Jr. You will find additional resources listed in the back of this book. For our present discussion, let's explore a few common matters that may stand in the way of us understanding that eating plant-based is in our best favor.

Some people are perplexed by the plant-based eating paradigm, believing that a meatless or dairy-less meal is somehow incomplete or that early humans were heavy meat-eaters, so we should predominantly follow their example. In Chapter 20, we will explore how ideas that lead to beliefs, whether true or not, spread through our society and impact our lives. From what we know thus far of historical data, early humans were hunter-gatherers, so their diet consisted of various plant stems, roots, fruits, leaves, tubers, nuts, seeds, insects and lean, fresh meat only when it could be captured. Evidence suggests that our roots (no pun intended) were more plant-based than the majority of us realize.[1,2] From a logical perspective, we must consider what food sources are easier to obtain: Is it easier to gather plants or hunt, trap, and kill animals? Geographical location must also be considered, as it influences dietary requirements and food availability. Industrialization aside, native cultures who reside in cold climates have always eaten diets rich in animal products, whereas native cultures who reside in warm climates have always eaten more plant products. The diets of some of our earliest ancestors may seem lucrative for many today, as can be seen by the popularity of The Paleo, Primal, or Caveman movements. The reasons behind this are two-fold. First, the grass always seems greener on the other side, and compared to The Standard American Diet, these are a huge step up. Many are frustrated and fed up, literally sick and tired of being sick and tired, so they will try anything and everything, even if it means going back to whatever we presume is square one. A diet that cuts out processed food will definitely do wonders! However, in our modern context, aside from any change in our bodies, our food is so different and has, itself, evolved as compared to what it was thousands or millions of years ago. Also, we do not really know for certain what it was like back then. Trying to piece it all together leaves us with more questions than answers. Rob Dunn, author and evolutionary biologist at North Carolina State University, sums it up really well:

"Eating some ancestral diet on its own will not make us healthy. Our ancestors did not eat diets perfectly in tune with their body. Rather, they took the best advantage of the foods around them they could in light of their bodies."[3]

The bottom line is that many dietary differences exist amidst different cultures and timelines, with respect to the plant to animal food ratio, and while the past can give us clues about the present, as the saying goes, "only look backward if that is the way you want to go." The ideal diet, if it exists, is the one that best meets our current needs. We must work within the context of our times, appropriately meeting and addressing our modern health, food, and planetary challenges. Today we have ample evidence, which you can explore at your leisure, linking diets high in animal products with all sorts of unfavorable effects. They simply are not good for us, nor are they good for our planet.

From the beginning, humans have thrived on a high-fiber (i.e. high-plant) diet. Even our most recent ancestors did not eat animal products in the proportions that are consumed by most in the industrialized world today. There is something innate within us that drives us to plants as our primary food source, unless we are under the influence of our processed food society. Many people do not realize that our animal-food-oriented mindset is actually quite recent, spurred heavily after the World Wars by the industrialization of foods in North America. We also know that whatever is made to seem scarce, limited, or rare seems to attract us all the more. For many centuries, animal foods were most often associated with the wealthy or those in power, considered a symbol of status. Today, if we are all eating like kings and queens, we're certainly paying a king's ransom for it.

When it comes to other animal foods, such as dairy, its emergence took place at about the same time as humans moved into agriculture, using grains, and having domestic animals, about 10,000 years ago. To this day, the majority of the world population cannot properly digest milk or milk products past infancy, and it is a myth to think we need dairy to survive, much less to thrive. Not only are we the only animal species who consumes milk past our weaning stage, but we also consume the milk of other animals, and today, that comes in the form of highly processed products.

In terms of our anatomy and physiology, some people argue the presence of some form of canine teeth, acid in the stomach, and the inability to break down cellulose as the reasons why we've been made to eat meat. However, it is not really a matter of whether or not we are or are not meant to eat meat. Yes, the human body is capable of digesting meat, even though our anatomy and physiology is very different from animals that are truly meant to eat meat. Looking at our closest animal relatives, the chimpanzees, it is worthy to note that their average diet consists of about 97 percent plant foods.[4] On such a diet, they build all the muscle mass they need, keeping naturally lean. However, this is also not about picking apart the details of human-chimpanzee characteristics or diets. What eating plant-based versus animal-based comes down to is a matter of quantity and quality of both. It is one thing to consume the meat of wild animals, animals that were raised and fed naturally, or dairy in its most natural form, and to consume these in small quantities infrequently; it is entirely another to eat meat from factory-farmed animals and processed dairy in large quantities daily. Beyond our anatomy, physiology, history, and evolution, the quality and quantity of animal products in our diet today is seriously working against us. The consequences of our actions do not require study; we have enough living, barely breathing proof walking around us. Our weight is suffering, our health is suffering, our mental and emotional wellbeing is suffering, and never before has society been so disconnected from the natural world.

All Plants Are Not Created Equal

If we are committed to maintaining the best health and weight, we must make the predominant amount of our daily foods come from whole, natural plants. Still, as mentioned earlier, while plants offer an array of unique health and nutrition benefits for us, all plant foods cannot be considered equal. Our plant foods must be in their most wholesome forms, and our diets should revolve around fruits and vegetables. Other plant foods to include in our daily diets include nuts, seeds, beans, legumes, grains, herbs, and spices. We will discuss each of their unique benefits and how to include them in ways that are best for our health in Part 2, when we cover specifically what to eat.

Fruits and vegetables, especially leafy greens, are, by far, the most beneficial plant foods for our health. Next are herbs and spices, which offer a wide variety of very powerful and concentrated nutrients, even when consumed in very small amounts. Next in line are beans and legumes, which should be eaten on a daily basis. They are packed with protein, fiber, and healthy carbohydrates, as well as vitamins, minerals, and phytonutrients. Nuts and seeds also offer many wonderful benefits for our health, one being that they are rich in healthy fats. We benefit most from eating these in small amounts, as part of our regular diet. Finally are grains, which offer some of the best sources of healthy carbohydrates and fuel for the body. However, we must be careful that our plant-based diet does not morph into a grain-based one. There are many wonderful, highly beneficial whole grains, like brown rice and oats, and seed grains, like quinoa and buckwheat, which we can enjoy on a regular basis. We just mustn't get caught up in processed grain products or let the bulk of our meals come from grains.

Practical Tips for Eating Plant-Based

To finish this section, here are some tips for making the best choices when it comes to eating healthy plant-based:

1. **Make vegetables, especially green leafy ones, a significant part of each meal.** The easiest and a very delicious way to start the day is with leafy greens in a green smoothie. Lunch and dinner can include abundant combinations of salads, soups, or steamed veggie dishes based on vegetables and/or leafy greens.

2. **Enjoy a variety of a few fruits each day.** While I don't want to restrict you to a certain number, my general advice is to enjoy between two to four servings of fruit daily. Some nutrition experts advise eating minimal fruits, while others promote fruit-based diets. Simply listen to your body and be flexible in this regard to account for any unique health needs, as well as seasonal considerations.

3. **Eat beans and legumes on a daily basis.** Cooked or fresh beans or legumes can be included as part of our regular diet in many unique, creative, delicious ways. Enjoy the immense variety as part of your homemade soups, chili, stews, salads, wraps, hummus, spreads, and dips.

4. **Enrich your meals with herbs and spices.** You can make your meals taste delicious, exploring the many unique flavor combinations possible with an

abundance of herbs and spices. Whether fresh or dried, use them liberally in your meals.

5. **Eat various raw nuts and seeds regularly.** These offer many valuable nutrients for our health. It is best to eat raw nuts that have not been roasted, and always choose plain varieties without any salt, seasoning, sugary coatings, or other processed additions. Nuts and seeds can be easily incorporated into most meals or eaten on their own as a snack, and they make amazing dips and creamy sauces. Nuts also make wonderful raw crusts for various healthy desserts, as well as delicious homemade nut milks.

6. **Go easy on the grains.** When you enjoy grains, focus on whole and unprocessed options. Incorporate them into some of your meals in modest amounts.

7. **Reduce consumption of animal products.** If you choose to eat meat, dairy, eggs, or seafood, make sure it is from the most natural, organic, and free-range sources. Your best option is a local farmer you trust. Animal products should never be the main part of the meal or the main food source of the day.

CHAPTER 4
Eating Acid-Alkaline Balanced

Acid-alkaline balanced eating, also known as alkaline eating, is an unfamiliar concept for many. However, once you discover how the acid-alkaline balance works, you will quickly realize that if you follow through with the eating guidelines I've shared with you thus far, you are most likely already eating well in this area. This balance is essential to optimally support our health, healing, and prevention, yet it is rarely mentioned in most nutrition dialogue. Luckily, entire books and other resources have been dedicated to this topic for those who wish to understand the intricate details of its biochemical nature. In this chapter, I will provide you with a practical summary to understand the basics of how this concept works. We'll start with a short review of chemistry basics, but there is no need to panic if chemistry wasn't your strong point in school! I plan to make it painless.

In chemistry, we are able to measure the pH (potential for Hydrogen) value of a substance using simple tools, mainly various indicators, to determine its pH (concentration of hydrogen ions). The pH scale ranges from zero to fourteen. This tells us whether a substance is acidic (less than seven), neutral (seven), or basic/alkaline (more than seven). This can also be done with the foods we eat. For example, using the pH paper indicator, one can quickly tell the pH value of tomatoes, strawberries, or milk, to know if they are acidic, neutral, or alkaline. When we are interested in eating acid-alkaline balanced, we are not interested in the pH properties of the food as it enters our body; rather, we are concerned with the pH properties of the *digested* components of the food. These are commonly referred to as the "ash," as we can compare our metabolism burning food for energy to a fire burning wood for energy, which produces ash residue. It is vital to understand this before we go any further. The original wood is neither physically nor chemically equivalent to its ash. Its properties have been transformed as it underwent the chemical burning reaction. When we apply this simple analogy to our food, we begin to understand why lemons may be acidic going into our bodies but actually have a very alkaline effect upon digestion. This is why, based on the acid-alkaline way of eating, we can classify all foods as either *acid-forming* or *alkaline-forming*.

Basics of the Acid-Alkaline Balance

Our bodies thrive on balance and operate best within narrowly controlled ranges of physical, chemical, and biochemical values. Examples of these include body temperature, blood pressure, blood sugar, heart rate, various mineral compositions, and blood pH. We know that if our bodies go outside these normal ranges, all sorts of dire consequences may result. Different fluids and organs need to operate within their own required pH as well, like our saliva, bile and urine, or our stomach, intestines, and skin. For the purpose of our discussion here, we will focus on our blood pH.

Normal blood pH must be maintained within the narrow range of 7.35 to 7.45 to ensure the proper functioning of metabolic processes and the delivery of the right amount of oxygen to tissues. In some literature, this range is even more narrowly referenced, with slight variations between arterial and venous blood. Regardless, the normal blood pH is slightly alkaline, and your body will do everything in its power to keep it that way. If your blood pH goes below that range, it results in acidosis (excess of acid in the blood), and if it goes above that range, it results in alkalosis (excess of base in the blood). Drastic shifts outside this range can be life threatening, while chronic, subtle shifts increase the likelihood of disease. A 2001 comprehensive study published in the *European Journal of Nutrition* has demonstrated that our modern, acid-producing diets create low-grade systemic metabolic acidosis in otherwise healthy adults, increasing with age and resulting in various health problems.[1]

Common factors that influence our blood pH include the gases we exchange (oxygen and carbon dioxide), exercise, stress, drugs, toxins, and our food. While dealing with these, our normal body functions and metabolism generate large quantities of acids that must be neutralized and/or eliminated to maintain the balance of our blood pH. To neutralize these acids, appropriate alkaline substances are required. Some of the richest of these include common minerals like calcium, magnesium, and potassium that are stored within our bones and ammonia-like substances, very alkaline, that are stored within our muscles. As you can imagine, if these are not readily available in our diet, it can result in bone and muscle loss. To support our optimal health, we must consume sufficient alkaline-forming foods that will work with, not against, the acid-alkaline balance, replenishing our stores accordingly. Our modern diet is unnaturally high in acid-forming foods, such as animal foods and grains, and unnaturally low in alkaline-forming foods, like vegetables and fruits. Thus, we are working against ourselves in two of the worst ways possible, setting the stage for all sorts of health problems.

To eliminate these acids effectively, the body's elimination channels must be working properly. The two main organs involved in the regulation of external acid-base balance are the lungs and the kidneys. The lungs are responsible for the uptake of oxygen and release of carbon dioxide, our respiratory acid. The kidneys are responsible for two key jobs in regard to regulating the pH, excreting metabolic acid waste, and reabsorbing bicarbonate, a highly valuable alkaline substance for the body. When the body is overwhelmed by acid waste or cannot expel it safely or quickly enough via the kidneys for any number of reasons, like kidney disease or diabetes, the body may begin to store the waste in fat tissue. Our fat cells are some of our most stable tissues, making them perfect storehouses for any toxins that would otherwise be disruptive or destructive to us. Chronic acidity is, therefore, associated with weight gain and a difficult time with weight loss. Those who alkalize their bodies appropriately commonly report successful results with weight loss. One of the best ways to help our lungs deal optimally with detoxing waste is to employ breathing exercises. Whether you incorporate these in yoga or meditation or just do them on your own, regular, conscious deep breathing is a valuable addition to optimally healthy lifestyle habits. One of the best ways to help optimize kidney function is to drink enough pure water throughout each day.

Diet has long been known to strongly affect the acid-base balance, yet we have just recently begun to look at the more detailed and profound nature of how it influences health maintenance and disease formation. In 2006, a professor of biochemistry and nutrition expert, Dr. Jurgen Vormann, organized "The Second International Acid-Base Symposium," which took place in Munich, Germany and brought together scientists from fifteen countries to examine the connections between diet, pH balance, and disease formation.[2] Their conclusions pointed to the fact that the modern diet is inadequate at satisfying the acid-alkaline balance, thus increasing the possibility of chronic, low-grade metabolic acidosis and, in the long run, disease.[3] The bulk of their research examined hormonal impairment and bone disease, namely osteoporosis. Other experts on this subject—like Dr. Susan E. Brown and Larry Trivieri Jr., authors of *The Acid-Alkaline Food Guide*, and Dr. Robert O. Young, author of *The pH Miracle*, and Dr. Theodore Baroody, author of *Alkalize or Die*—have linked chronic, low-grade acidosis (due to an acidic lifestyle) to inflammation, oxidative stress, heart disease, diabetes, cancer, kidney stones, kidney disease, muscle loss/deterioration, migraines, diminished immunity, accelerated aging, blood pressure irregularities, and problems regulating weight. In 2011, a review of some of the recent literature on the connection between an alkaline diet and various disease was conducted and published in the *Journal of Environmental and Public Health*, further substantiating many of these links.[4] Another consequence, and part of the cause of these imbalances, are various nutrient deficiencies related to the body constantly having to work to restore its balance. If all this is not bad enough, most disease-causing or problematic micro-organisms, like candida, thrive in a polluted, acidic system. Cellular acidosis is believed to be a leading factor in almost all chronic diseases.

How Do We Eat Alkaline?

While the acid-alkaline way of eating seems like a new idea to many people, including most conventional healthcare providers, it is not really a new concept at all. In fact, it dates back thousands of years, to ancient Indian Ayurvedic tradition and Chinese medicine. There were also pioneers of such thinking here in the West, beginning in the 1900s with Drs. William Howard Hay, MD and Arthur C. Guyton, MD, leading authorities on the acid-alkaline health balance and its correlation to excess weight and disease formation. In 1931, biochemist Otto Heinrich Warburg, one of the twentieth century's leading cell biologists, received The Nobel Prize in Physiology or Medicine "for his discovery of the nature and mode of action of the respiratory enzyme," related to his cancer research. His discoveries included that the root cause of cancer is too much acidity in the body and not enough oxygen; two sides of the same coin. As Dr. Gabriel Cousens, MD shares in his book *Spiritual Nutrition*, poor diet contributes to a form of oxygen stress by generating an excess of hydrogen ions

(H+), acidity in the system, which deplete oxygen by combining with it to create water. Today, acid-alkaline balance is most notably understood and utilized to aid healing, reverse disease, and prevent sickness, particularly by those in the alternative or natural health fields, including naturopathic doctors.

Recall that all foods can be classified as acid-forming or alkaline-forming. Researchers have gone even further in their classification, stating that some foods are highly, moderately, or mildly acidifying, where as others are mildly, moderately, or highly alkalizing. You can look up all sorts of colored acid-alkaline food charts online to help you determine exactly which foods are acidifying and which are alkalizing and to what degree. These are helpful at the start, but don't get caught up in picking apart the details; it is not meant to be difficult. You may note that there are slight variations between sources when it comes to some specific food ratings, but the general food pattern is consistent. Ultimately, to eat acid-alkaline balanced, you need about three-quarters (75 to 80 percent) of your daily food to come from alkaline-forming foods and about one-quarter (20 to 25 percent) to come from acid-forming foods. If we are in optimal shape, meaning that our weight is ideal and we are not suffering from any obvious health conditions, we can perhaps afford to eat about 60 to 40 percent alkaline-to-acid-forming foods, but it is always to our advantage to aim for the higher alkaline composition. The current dietary practices of the majority are very much the reverse of this, with people eating only about 20 to 40 percent alkaline-forming foods and 60 to 80 percent acid-forming foods. In light of this, our weight and disease statistics should come as no surprise. It is also important to note that for optimal health's sake, we should not eat completely alkaline. While your body does require a high supply of alkaline-forming foods, it also needs some acid-forming foods.

To eat in a way that supports our acid-alkaline balance, we need to base our diets on vegetables, namely leafy greens, and fruits. These are the most powerful alkaline-forming foods. The reason for this is twofold. First, they don't produce much acidic ash, and second, they are rich in alkaline-forming minerals like potassium, calcium, and magnesium. Speaking of potassium, it appears to be drastically lacking in our diets today, and to make matters worse, it is overshadowed by the amount of sodium in our diets. Research suggests that our evolutionary diets had a ratio of about 10:1 potassium to sodium; today, we are eating about 1:3 potassium to sodium.[5] Aside from increasing alkaline-forming foods, we need to reduce the amount of acid-forming foods, namely animal products (meat, dairy, eggs), grains, sugar, salt, coffee, alcohol, and soda. The common byproducts of acid-forming foods are sulfuric acid, commonly found in animal protein, phosphoric acid, commonly found in soda, and uric acid, commonly found in meat. We also need to be mindful of any non-food items that affect our bodies, such as prescription medication, stress and over-strenuous exercise, which can all further disrupt our pH balance. Given all that you have learned, it may cross your mind that something like dairy, which we equate with high calcium amounts, might actually be an excellent food with which to support the acid-alkaline balance. Yet common, pasteurized dairy is acid-forming. Recall why fruits and vegetables were mentioned above as being the top choices. It is advantageous to bring in some alkalizing benefits, but if the food is highly acidifying, the alkalizing substances like calcium will be used to offset the effects of this imbalance, leaving little benefit for us, if any at all. This is part of the reason why, despite being some of the highest consumers of dairy, North Americans are plagued with some of the worst bone health on the planet.

Lack of sufficient fruits and vegetables and high reliance on animal products are, unfortunately, not our only problems. We also have a high reliance on grains, and, worse yet, on processed and refined ones in particular. Whether whole or refined, though, most grains are acidifying for our body. This is why, as already mentioned, we should not allow the bulk of our meals or diet to be based on grains. There are degrees of how acid-forming a particular grain is, with processed/refined/floured grains being the worst and whole-seed grains, like quinoa or buckwheat, being the best. Corn and wheat are specifically amongst the most highly acid-producing grains. According to Michael Pollan, author of *In Defense of Food*, corn, soy, and wheat currently make up about 67 percent of the average person's diet in the U.S. Corn has infiltrated almost every processed food in our grocery stores today, including meat. It is a major food source for factory-farmed animals, despite being unnatural and unhealthy for them.

Refined sugar and salt are also highly acidifying, and they contribute, in large part, to our common health and weight problems. This is another convincing reason to avoid processed food, as all of it is an abundant source of both. Neither of these two substances support healing, prevention, or optimal weight and health. We will address healthier alternatives to each in Chapter 14, but for the time being, choosing natural salts like unrefined sea or Himalayan salt, which contain many alkaline-producing minerals, is a much better way to go. The same highly acidifying effects go for coffee, soda, juice beverages, and alcohol, which will be further explained in Chapter 13.

There are ways to assess your personal levels of acidity. The best method is to consult with a competent naturopathic doctor who has the right diagnostic tools. This is a good idea, especially if you are already suffering from any health conditions that you would like to heal naturally. You can also experiment yourself with narrow range pH strips for the saliva and urine, which you can easily find at your local health food store. The best way to use these is to take several readings throughout the day, starting upon waking and keeping a record for a few weeks to see how things change and progress as you modify your dietary habits. Regardless of whether you do any testing or not, your body will likely speak to you loud and clear as you alkalize it, giving you the most substantial proof that you are moving in the right direction.

Practical Tips for Eating Alkaline

To finish this section, here are some tips for making the best choices when it comes to eating within a healthy acid-alkaline range:

1. **Eat a rich amount of dark, leafy greens each day.** Top choices include kale, collard greens, Swiss chard, spinach, bok choy, and romaine lettuce. Ideally, a good portion of leafy greens should be included with at least two, if not all three of our daily meals. Mornings are best started with green smoothies, lunches can be based on green salads, and dinners can include a variety of steam or stir-fried vegetable and leafy green options.

2. **Eat a diet based on vegetables and fruits.** The emphasis, as we mentioned in Chapter 3, should always be on vegetables, but fruits are also a necessary addition to our daily diet. Enjoy a variety of colorful fruits and vegetables regularly.

3. **If eating meat, eat wholesome, lean, organic meat only.** Meat products from such sources are less problematic than conventional, factory-farmed meat and processed meat products. They also offer different nutrient profiles and

tend to be less acidifying on the body. If eaten at all, meat should be consumed infrequently and in small portions, from local, free-range, pasture/grass-fed, organic sources only.

4. **Reduce your overall grain consumption and consume real, whole grains.** Keep evolving your dietary habits toward a complete elimination of processed grain products from your diet, including most whole-grain versions of breads, buns, cereals, crackers, bagels, pitas, and pastas. These commonly contain many problematic ingredients and additives that go above and beyond the refined grain issues. Avoid commercial cakes, cookies, doughnuts, and other white flour pastry items. When you do eat grains, eat real, whole grains like brown rice, buckwheat, quinoa, amaranth and millet, balanced in your meals with sufficient vegetables.

5. **Reduce or entirely avoid dairy.** We have ample evidence today that dairy does not lead to optimal bone health; in fact, it may actually work against your bone health. Processed, pasteurized milk, cheese, and yogurt should be avoided entirely. For any dairy needs you may have, source out organic, unflavored, naturally fermented, and possibly raw, wholesome options for infrequent consumption.

6. **Avoid acid-forming beverages.** Key culprits are coffee, soda, pasteurized juices, energy drinks, caffeinated tea, and alcohol. The majority of these offer nothing more than empty calories, various synthetic ingredients, sugars, and lots of health problems. Replace destructive beverages with pure water, and squeeze in fresh lemon or lime juice for an added boost of alkalizing benefits, as may be desired.

7. **Avoid processed/refined sugars, and most isolated sweeteners.** Refined sugar, whether white or brown, processed sugar derivatives, artificial sweeteners, and sugary snacks are all detrimental to your health. Refined and isolated sugars negatively affect nearly all areas of the body, including oral, bone, digestive, cardiovascular, and even emotional health. Replace sugary snacks with fresh or dried fruit and other wholesome snacks.

8. **Avoid commercial condiments.** Ketchup, mayonnaise, salad dressings, and other sauces and dips are full of refined sugar, salt, and additives,

contributing both unnecessary calories and acidifying properties to your meals. When a particular meal calls for some condiment-like addition, create your own sauces, dips, and dressings with real, wholesome, ingredients like extra virgin olive oil, lemon or lime juice, apple cider vinegar, herbs, spices, nuts, seeds, ginger, onion, and garlic.

9. **Replace your salt and reduce overall intake.** At home, replace refined salt with unrefined sea salt or Himalayan salt, and use it sparingly in your meals. Avoid or limit refined salt and high sodium by avoiding processed food altogether.

CHAPTER 5
Eating Raw

Eating raw means eating food in its most natural form. There is no doubt that we have gained a lot, evolutionarily speaking, by incorporating the practice of cooking our food. It has improved palatability, bioavailability, and safety. However, like many other things in life, we have also taken this practice to extremes, going out of balance and moving away from Mother Nature's most optimized method of delivery. As such, we are sacrificing a lot of nutritional integrity and subjecting ourselves to various imbalances and health disadvantages. Thus, the next way to optimize our eating for optimal health, weight, healing, and prevention is to consume a large portion of our food raw.

You may have heard of the raw food movement or the popularity of raw food diets. While this discussion borders on the foundation of those paradigms, it is not about becoming a raw foodist, aiming to eat 100 percent raw. Just like with plant-based and alkaline-based eating, the solution is to eat the *majority* of your food, around 75 percent (three-quarters), in its most natural form. Again, if you are following with the guidelines presented thus far, this should be easy and intuitive for you.

Why Raw?

Raw foods are created and packaged with Mother Nature's intelligence in mind. While we may not yet fully understand the reasons behind it all, it is in our best interest to respect the process and state of the final product. The main reason to eat raw is to preserve and take advantage of food's original nutritional integrity in the fullest way possible. Whole, natural plant foods, as we already covered, are full of vital nutrients like vitamins, minerals, phytonutrients, and antioxidants, many of which are sensitive to heat and oxidation or are water-soluble and easily lost. Experts and research concur that raw fruits and vegetables offer the highest blood levels of cancer-protective nutrients and more protection than any other foods, including cooked plant foods.[1]

Another important characteristic of raw foods, specifically raw plant foods, are *enzymes*. These are composed of amino acids, which are created and secreted by your body. They enable the biological processes necessary for optimal body functions, like building materials, breaking down materials, circulating nutrients, eliminating waste, and a myriad of others. There are thousands of enzymes that we know of, but experts estimate there may be tens of thousands we have yet to discover. The three categories of enzymes include: *metabolic, digestive,* and *food enzymes*. Metabolic enzymes work within your cells, digestive enzymes work outside your cells, helping to break down food, and food enzymes come from our food. Physician, researcher, and pioneer in enzyme research, Dr. Edward Howell, dedicated much of his life to studying enzymes and their connection to our health and disease creation. He, like many other experts, believed the enzymes naturally present in raw foods are of significant help in digesting the foods themselves; that cooking destroys enzymes, forcing the body to rely on its own enzymes; and that this reliance on enzymes due to high cooked-food diets decreases our digestive potential as we age. The latter contributes to the increased digestive troubles that are so commonly experienced, especially in our later years. Today, Dr. Howell's theories are debated, and it is clear that more research must be done in this area before we will understand it properly or thoroughly. However, there is no debating the fact that cooking above certain temperatures destroys enzymes. These compounds are very heat sensitive and one of the reasons why high fevers are dangerous to us, since our bodies rely on enzymes for so many critical reactions. The question that remains is to what degree are the enzymes naturally found in raw foods protective and beneficial for us.

The human body and its enzymes function best within the range of 35 to 40 degrees Celsius or 95 to 104 degrees Fahrenheit, with 36.6 degrees Celsius and 98 degrees Fahrenheit being our average, normal body temperature. Food enzymes are destroyed at temperatures above the range of 46 to 48 degrees Celsius (115 to 118 degrees Fahrenheit). When we heat natural, living foods too much, we denature the enzymes, changing both their shape and function and disabling them from performing the necessary task. Chronic loss of these functions over the years is believed to be taxing on the digestive system, to the point that, as we age, many people are rendered unable to properly digest certain foods. The resulting enzyme deficiency, sometimes referred to as *cellular enzyme exhaustion*, can lead to poor digestion, poor nutrient absorption, and a variety of gastrointestinal problems, including constipation, diarrhea, bloating, cramping, flatulence, belching, heartburn, and acid reflux. Enzyme supplements can be used to aid digestion, but the whole point of our discussion is that we should do things as naturally as possible and allow our food to offer the possible healing, prevention, and optimal health we seek.

From an evolutionary perspective, like all other animals, human beings have consumed foods in raw form, especially plant foods. The move to more cooked food appeared to be a beneficial step for our ancestors, who were prone to food scarcity; cooked foods do provide more calories than their raw counterparts. The more processed a food is, whether cooked at home or in a factory, the more calories are available to us, as compared to food in its natural, raw state.[2] Take carrots, for example. Your body will get far more calories from canned or cooked carrots than the same amount of raw. Generally speaking, the more natural the food and the more work the body needs to do to digest it, the less of its maximum potential of calories we get. As such, raw fruits and vegetables are not just better for our health; they are also really helpful in maintaining a healthy weight. While our ancestors might have benefitted from the extra calories, due to decreased food security and increased physical activity, today, our health and weight are most likely to benefit from going back to food's natural, raw form.

Cooked foods also appear to cause inflammation and oxidative stress. Without getting into too many nitty-gritty details, a reaction in our body, *glycation*, involves the joining of a carbohydrate to a protein without the use of an enzyme. This results in the production of compounds called *advanced glycation end products* (AGEs), which appear to have a negative impact on our health and increase as we age. When it comes to our food, it can be both a source of extrinsic AGEs and something that influences the creation of intrinsic AGEs. Foods subjected to high or prolonged temperatures through cooking practices like frying or grilling, including some plants but mostly high-protein, high-fat animal foods, produce AGEs. So what exactly is the problem with AGEs? Research has shown a direct association between dietary AGE intake and inflammation, leading to chronic disease.[3] Although more research is still needed to fully understand the impacts of dietary AGEs, studies continue to link increased AGEs with the formation of chronic diseases such as cardiovascular disease, Type 2 diabetes, Alzheimer's, arthritis, and kidney disease, as well as negatively impacting longevity.[4,5] To decrease our risk of AGE-related damage, we must eat more foods in their natural (raw) state, decrease the heat intensity and duration of any cooking we do, and increase our intake of antioxidants, which can repair some of the damage caused by AGEs.

Finally, foods cooked under high or prolonged heat, especially when it discolors the food with shades of brown or black, contain carcinogenic compounds. This holds true for most starches and animal products, that are subjected to baking, grilling, and barbecuing. Under high heat, *acrylamide* forms in high-carbohydrate, low-protein foods. This substance is most common in potatoes, especially French fries or chips. In animal products, high heat results in the formation of *heterocyclic amines*, which we will discuss more in Chapter 12. While it is not a huge problem to eat a few of these foods in your lifetime, it becomes a big deal when such foods are part of your regular diet.

You may be wondering about claims you've heard about cooked food being easier to digest and even higher in some nutrients. Generally speaking, these assumptions are true. Heat and various forms of food processing tend to break down the tough cell walls of plants, making the food easier for us to digest. However, this can work both for and against us, as we have touched upon already. We can improve digestibility by blending food rather than cooking it, which would prove more beneficial from a nutrient perspective. It is also one of the reasons why green smoothies are an excellent addition to our diet. As for increased nutrient values, we may indeed win some in cooking, but we will always lose some, and the loss appears greater than any gain that results. Even for tomatoes, which are most commonly cited as having improved lycopene (a phytonutrient) concentration upon cooking, blending them appears to unlock just as much or similar amounts of lycopene, according to raw food and nutrition expert David Wolfe. Ultimately, there are two important things we should remember: Nutrients, like the lycopene in tomatoes, are still there and available to us in the food's raw form, and second, we do not have to consume *everything* raw. A raw way of eating can be much more flexible than most people think. If you are not a fan of raw broccoli, for example, you can lightly steam it and still benefit from the nutrients it naturally contains.

Finally, if we steer a little in the direction of a more metaphysical nature, we bring to our awareness the concept of food's actual living energy. We will discuss this a little in Chapter 20 and talk about how it relates to us, but basically, all living things have a life force, commonly referred to as *chi* or *qi*. It is the central underlying principle of Traditional Chinese Medicine, but it crosses over to many other disciplines, including quantum science. Fresh, living, whole plant foods have a more powerful life force than any processed plant foods. This is why processed or heavily cooked food is referred to as "dead food"; it has lost most of its life energy, if not all of it. Meat, in this regard, speaks for itself. Although it may sound a little farfetched for some of us, the deeper you go on your holistic and personal evolution journey, the more this will make sense and be of importance to you. The concept is not that abstract either, as we can actually see and measure this bioelectrical energy—the life force of living things—using a tool like Kirlian photography. Some people can also easily feel the energy, and several holistic therapies are based on the movement of energy. I personally love the following saying that sums up this topic really well: "Living bodies require living foods".

How to Eat Raw

From everything we have covered and learned thus far, the bulk of our food should consist of vegetables, leafy greens, and fruits in their whole, natural forms. This pretty much automatically guarantees them for us in their raw forms. As for other foods, the rule of thumb is as follows: Without the need to measure or calculate anything, simply focus on cooking food at the lowest temperatures and for the shortest periods of time possible. Let's examine some of our foods in more detail.

In terms of nuts, seeds, grains, beans, and legumes, the ideal way to prepare and consume most of them is to soak and/or sprout them. Soaking literally makes the seed come alive, out of its dormancy, to prepare for growing of a new plant. For our purposes, it ensures that the foods not only maintain their optimal enzyme and nutrient levels but even increase them. The process of soaking/sprouting neutralizes or inactivates digestive inhibitors that many of these foods contain, thereby rendering more nutrients available to us. Grains and beans contain some enzyme inhibitors and a substance known as *phytic acid*, which can combine with iron, calcium, magnesium, copper, and zinc in the intestinal tract, blocking their absorption. Sprouting or even just soaking these foods with or without cooking, neutralizes these compounds. It is worthy to add that soaked/sprouted nuts, seeds, grains, and beans also tend to have a more alkalizing, less acidifying effect on our bodies, thereby favorably supporting the acid-alkaline balance. Ancient societies and many people to this day only eat grains that have been soaked, sprouted, or fermented for optimal digestion and health benefits. It is also noteworthy that many people who have a hard time tolerating grains have a completely different and positive, digestive reaction to grains that have been soaked or sprouted. Many grocery stores and local farmers' markets today sell all sorts of sprouts that can be easily incorporated in our regular diets, as well as soaked, sprouted, flourless, whole grain, and legume breads.

The most important thing for optimal health, healing, and prevention is to avoid highly cooked or processed foods. Likewise, reheating foods many times, as in the case of leftovers, should be minimized or avoided; each time you subject that food to more heat, you lose more of its nutritional and healing value. In our often-rushed, fast-paced lives, we always seem to be struggling for time and looking for ways to cut corners. However, while you can optimize your lifestyle in many ways to make it more efficient, it should never be at the expense of your food and proper nutrition. When we make time for nourishing and healing our bodies properly, we ensure that the time we do have will be spent in the best of health.

What About Raw Animal Foods?

Technically, the healthiest way to eat animal foods is raw. I know this is not what you wanted to hear; however, one of the reasons for this, aside from any nutrient loss during heat application, is that they are dense in protein. As you may recall from our enzyme discussion, amino acids, which make up protein, become denatured by high heat, amongst other factors. This change in shape and function can render the protein less available for us, but it can also lead to the risk and intensity of chronic diseases linked with inflammation. The latter is related to the AGEs and carcinogenic heterocyclic amines we discussed earlier. Pasteurized dairy is also associated with a whole slew of problems, from nutrient deficiencies to troubles for our health. Fried foods, including eggs, can also be hard on the liver. Of course, the other side of the coin is not without its own risks. By eating raw animal products, we expose ourselves to various serious bacterial risks and infections.

Please understand that I am, in no way, advocating or advising that you eat raw animal products. This is a very sensitive personal choice that will require a thorough consideration of various tradeoffs. If you are interested in keeping various animal products in your diet, you should do more research on this topic and decide what is right for you, your health, and your weight. Even today, some cultures frequently consume specially marinated raw meat, and some health experts insist that if you consume milk or eggs, they should only be raw. However, just as there are benefits to these, there are also inherent risks. The first step to reduce these risks is to drastically reduce the amount of animal products in your diet. If you are going to eat cooked animal foods, avoid frying, grilling, broiling, or barbecuing them. Aside from the tips below, we will cover more about eating animal products in the safest way possible in Chapter 12.

Practical Tips for Eating Raw

To finish this section, here are some tips for making the best choices for healthy, safe raw eating:

1. **Eat the majority of your fruits and vegetables raw.** Whether gently steamed or entirely raw, this is the most beneficial way to consume these foods. These foods have the most to offer and the most to lose, so increase their benefits by preserving their nutritional integrity.

2. **Eat raw nuts and seeds.** Avoid all roasted nuts and seeds. Their healthy fats and protein are denatured by the heat and may end up working against us. Only source out and consume raw nuts and seeds. You can improve the digestibility of most nuts and seeds by soaking them for a few hours or even sprouting them.

3. **Try sprouting some grains and beans.** Any dry beans you use, and even some grains, should be soaked overnight. Typically, anywhere from twelve to twenty-four hours of soaking is common prior to cooking. Do try,

however, to experiment with sprouting some grains and beans, or enjoy sprouts that you can easily access from your stores or farmers' markets.

4. **Boil your meats and steam your fish, instead of frying, grilling, barbecuing, or roasting them.** Avoid exposing animal flesh (meat and seafood) to high and prolonged temperatures. Cook up to the point that is needed for your personal safety, but avoid creating any brown or black buildup on meat. Steaming fish and boiling meats is a healthier way to consume them.

5. **Avoid dairy altogether or consider raw dairy.** If you are going to keep dairy in your diet, especially milk, look for local, organic farmers who can provide high-quality raw milk. This is the most nutritious way to consume milk of another species; it still contains all the rich vitamins, minerals, raw proteins, and other nutrients that are otherwise stripped out or destroyed during the pasteurization process.

6. **Avoid baking and browning of carbohydrate-rich foods, and go for raw desserts.** There are numerous raw, whole-food, plant-based desserts, some of which I will share with you in this book. These can satisfy your sweet tooth, providing benefits without the downsides. They are nutrient-dense and highly delicious! From raw brownies and raw cheesecakes (dairy-free) to raw cookies and bars of all sorts, there is something to please everyone. Enjoy exploring the amazing variety of possibilities. As for breads and similar products, remember that we want to reduce our reliance on processed grains altogether, but you can occasionally enjoy some wholesome, flourless sprouted grain and legume breads or wraps, commonly labeled as Ezekiel bread, or high-quality wholesome sourdough ones.

CHAPTER 6
Eating Organic

Eating organic means eating foods that have been grown or farmed according to traditional methods, without synthetic fertilizers, chemical pesticides, or genetic modification. For millennia, we were able to depend on a vast variety of wild plant foods, and we later found favorable and natural ways to cultivate them. However, in the last 200 years, more specifically since the early 1900s, that natural landscape of food production has drastically changed. One of the reasons behind this was our rapidly expanding human population; another reason was the industrialization of family farms, which led to factory farming and monocultures. Financial profit became our biggest goal, and we used our technology to control the parts of nature we felt were working against it. It didn't take long, though, merely a few decades, for us to begin seeing the consequences of our actions. Nature does not operate based on profit; its focus is on balance, and when we disrupt that balance, we put into motion repercussions that disrupt our own balance.

Our discussion of how to eat would be incomplete if we did not consider modern food production challenges that pose various threats to our health and wellbeing. The application of diverse and extensive chemical pesticides and synthetic fertilizers to our plant foods, as well as unnatural feed, hormones, and drugs injected and fed to our animal foods, are all historically novel phenomena. Yet nowadays, organic is the exception rather than the rule, and we have to be convinced to eat organically, as if it is some sort of fad diet someone is trying to sell rather than the natural way that is most in alignment with the health of our body and planet. It is not a fad, though, and there is no getting away from it or trying to ignore it. To support our body for optimal health and weight, healing, and prevention, we need to make sure our food is as natural, nutrient-dense, and chemical-free as possible. This increases its healing and health-optimizing properties and equips us with a stronger foundation from which to thrive.

Why Eat Organic?

When food is grown according to certified or honest organic farming methods, it does not have hormones, antibiotics, synthetic fertilizers and pesticides, or genetically modified organisms added to it. There are four main reasons why we should eat organic for optimal health, weight, healing, and prevention:

1. Reduced chemical exposure and toxin loads

2. Avoidance of genetically modified organisms (GMOs)

3. Higher nutrient composition

4. Better taste

In addition to these positive aspects, organic foods are also more ecologically friendly and environmentally sustainable, though these issues are outside the scope of this book. If you would like to learn more about these benefits, there are plenty of other resources that focus specifically on them.

Within the realm of what we are discussing here, the first reason to eat organic is that we simply should not put any more chemicals in our system, especially those that come from the very things that are supposed to aid our health and prevent disease. Many of the chemicals used for growing our food are, for lack of a better word, toxic to us. Perhaps you think that if they were so bad, they would not be allowed, but I encourage you to recall my points from earlier chapters about the importance of taking personal accountability. Governments and corporations have their own priorities, agendas, and profit margins; you need to and deserve to have your own priorities met. It is usually only after a synthetic substance has shown considerable and directly linked harm that governing bodies even begin to limit its use or enforce guidelines for its use. Some of the chemicals that are liberally sprayed or applied to our food display carcinogenic and neurotoxic properties, not to mention are suspected to cause allergies and hormonal imbalances, among many other problems. Our governments and citizens do not take these chemicals seriously enough, partly because when a disease or condition develops, it is almost impossible to trace it back to one specific chemical source. This is one of the reasons why there are not more bans on chemical substances and ingredients, though they do tend to replace one pesticide with another if too many problems begin to surface; in essence swapping one poison for another. Ironically, our society invests so much money and time in detox programs, yet we do not seem to want to tackle this problem at the root level of prevention. The easiest way to free our bodies of chemicals is to not put them there in the first place.

We can talk a lot about the wide array of pesticides and their various negative health effects, but I don't want to turn this discussion into a drawn-out persuasion more than it already needs to be. Every time we eat conventionally grown produce, we subject ourselves to pesticides, and none of those pesticides belong in our bodies, period. As Chuck Benbrook, a research professor at the Center for Sustaining Agriculture and Natural Resources at Washington State University shares in the book *Toxin Toxout*, by Bruce Lourie and Rick Smith, by choosing organic, we lower the risks associated with pesticides approximately eighty-fold. Unfortunately, it may no longer be possible to find food that is 100 percent pesticide-free, due to the infiltration of chemicals to most parts of our planet. Pesticide residues are a grim reality in our chemically inundated world, even for organic food. Nevertheless, we can and should have a huge say in whether or not we're willing to add or keep toxins out of our bodies. As demonstrated by the research presented and experiment conducted in *Toxin Toxout*, an organic diet provides almost immediate benefits, reducing the body's pesticide level output and input.

Our fruits and vegetables, our most valuable and prized food sources, are some of the most vulnerable targets if they are non-organic. Some are heavily sprayed, and many retain their pesticide application. Unlike nuts or fruits that have hard shells or thick peels, most produce has no natural shield from the assaulting pesticides, so we ingest whatever is retained on and inside them. To learn how to be a smart consumer when it comes to which produce should only be consumed in its organic form and which you can afford to buy from conventional sources, I recommend *EWG's Shopper's Guide to Pesticides in Produce*. Each year, the Environmental Working Group releases an annual report of the worst and best choices in produce, specifically focusing on pesticides, and compiles it in this free and very helpful guide.

EWG's Shopper's Guide to Pesticides in Produce
www.ewg.org/foodnews

Animal foods have their own problems when they are not derived from organic sources; in many ways, these can be even more serious. The first problem is the feed given to the animals, which includes pesticide-sprayed crops and/or genetically modified crops. Because animals are higher up on the food chain, and due to their significant fat composition as compared to plants, toxins readily accumulate in their tissues, just as they do in ours. Thus, when you eat conventional animal foods, you are also consuming the toxins that have accumulated in that animal's body. It is not healthy for us to have toxins in our bodies, and it is not healthy for animals to harbor them either, so we must consider the quality of the meat, eggs, or milk that come from such animals. To add to all this, factory-farmed and some independently farmed animals are routinely given various drugs, including antibiotics and hormones. This further imbalances their health and, consequently, the quality of the product you will ultimately ingest.

When it comes to GMOs, the *Grocery Manufacturers of America* estimate that between 70 to 75 percent of all processed foods available in U.S. grocery stores may contain ingredients from genetically engineered plants. It is widely known that corn, soy, and canola are the most susceptible to genetic engineering today. Many other foods are undergoing experimentations or are already being sold with some form of genetic modification. Examples include alfalfa, salmon, potatoes, tomatoes, squash, and papaya. The FDA and other governing bodies continue to insist that genetically modified foods are "substantially equivalent to unmodified" and "pose no inherent safety risk," but emerging studies are proving otherwise. A 2011 paper published in *Environmental Science Europe* reviewed nineteen animal studies, revealing that genetically modified foods may damage the immune system and organs, causing infertility, insulin deregulation, increased mortality, accelerated aging, and potential precancerous cell growth, with the liver and kidneys being most affected.[1] Many European countries and others in the world want nothing to do with genetically modified (GM) foods, but Canada and the United States continue to pacify any risks associated with them. The liver and kidney connection alone should make us tune in to the fact that there appears to be some food toxicity present when it comes to consuming GM foods. Most of us are unaware that many genetically modified crops are still treated with pesticides, smacking all who eat them with a double-whammy of problems.

The good news is that we, as consumers, are both waking up and speaking up. The wave of GMO labeling initiatives sweeping across the globe speaks for itself, as do the millions of dollars invested by biotech companies to prevent those labeling laws from passing. Ingredients and nutrition fact labeling is in place to help us make good choices. As such, there should be no question that genetically modified organisms should be properly labeled, yet the companies are fighting with everything they've got to prevent this from happening, claiming that it will unnecessarily scare consumers away from purchasing the food. The truth is that they are correct, with the exception of the "unnecessarily" part. When we engineer the DNA of one species with the DNA of another, we create substances that are completely foreign to our bodies and their genetic and biochemical understanding of our food. It is naïve to think that these substances will have no noticeable and profound impact on us and on the rest of nature. Ultimately, the politics of GMOs run far and wide, and it is clear that they are not going away anytime soon. While they claim otherwise, they are not going to end world hunger, nor will they solve our food production challenges, as many would like us to believe. Therefore, our best action as consumers is to educate ourselves about them and understand that, when given a choice, we should ultimately side with Mother Nature. After all, she will ultimately have the final say.

When it comes to a higher nutrient composition of organic foods, it appears the jury is still out on the issue, though, an increasing number of scientific studies are reporting significant, beneficial results. For example, a 2003 study published in the *Journal of Agricultural and Food Chemistry* found that organically grown berries and corn contained 58 percent more of a certain antioxidant and up to 52 percent higher levels of Vitamin C than those conventionally grown.[2] Other studies, report organic foods have higher levels of various vitamins, minerals, antioxidants, and phytonutrients in the specific foods tested, as compared to conventional counterparts.[3] Regardless, we don't have to wait for some study to prove to us that organic food is better for us; it just takes some simple gardening knowledge to understand why they are. The quality of the plant and its fruit is highly dependent on the quality of the soil. Rich, fertile, organic soils will naturally produce crops that are higher in quality than crops harvested from nutritionally depleted soils. Of course today, most conventional produce is grown with ample synthetic fertilizers that spike the nutrient levels of the soil, but this is not a natural process, and it will never be able to compete with nature's own regulation systems. Simply put, synthetic nutrients are not the same as natural or integral nutrients. We will discuss this further in Chapter 16, when we talk about supplements and why they do not hold all the answers for us either. Sure, you may get some of the biggest and best-looking fruits and vegetables from plants treated with synthetic fertilizers, but don't be fooled by external appearances. Truly, when it comes to your food and your health, it's what's on the inside that counts.

While taste or flavor does not necessarily influence our health, it often influences how much we will enjoy our food. Rich, natural flavors can also be indicative of fresher, more nutritious food. Organic food, especially produce, has been noted to taste better. You and I can easily do a taste test ourselves, trying different organic foods next to their conventionally grown counterparts. All of our taste buds may detect flavors slightly different, but the differences will be obvious to each of us personally. A two-year study led by John Reganold of Washington State University provided side-by-side comparisons of organic and conventional strawberry farms. The organic farms produced higher quality fruit in terms of flavor and several nutrient levels, while promoting healthier and more genetically diverse soils.[4] I have personally tried many organic and conventionally grown fruits and vegetables, and I can frequently tell whether they are organic or not, simply based on taste and appearance. I have my own organic food garden, and I can attest, with enthusiastic certainty, that it yields some of the best-tasting produce I have ever eaten. Yes, organic matters, but local and fresh matter as well—not only when it comes to flavor but for nutrient integrity as well.

Examining the Excuses Opposing Organic

As I mentioned, many people almost have to have their arm twisted today when it comes to organics, and even then, some of us come up with all sorts of reasons to oppose it, as if it is something bad for us. This is somewhat understandable, especially since it often comes down to a financial choice. Let's face it: If something costs more, we need to be convinced that it really is worth it. Hopefully, the worth of it is taking on some clarity for you, since you have read this far. We always have a choice: We can invest in prevention or invest in treatment. Personally, I prefer prevention. While most organic, whole foods still cost slightly to significantly more than their non-organic counterparts, there are various ways to remedy this issue. First, it comes down to priorities. Many of us have no problem buying a case of beer, an overpriced cup of gourmet latte, or a lotto ticket regularly, yet if we are asked to pay just one dollar more for organic broccoli, it is a big problem. I fully understand that some people can barely afford fresh produce at all, let alone organic, but that is a whole other story. For the purpose of our discussion, simply be honest with yourself and mindful about how you choose to use your money. Every choice you make will directly impact you and your world and the society we all contribute to. Organics continue to be more readily available and abundant and continue to come down in price because more of us are choosing them, thus positively affecting societal change.

Furthermore, it is important to acknowledge that not every organic food item is more expensive. Some cost about the same, some go on sale, and some are even cheaper than conventionally grown foods. Explore the organic sections at your local grocery store regularly, as prices fluctuate. We can also work the system to our advantage by eating seasonally. Yes, organic strawberries can cost six dollars per pound in the winter, as opposed to half that in the summer, but we don't need to eat them in the winter. Learning to eat seasonally can be of great benefit to our health and our wallets. Seek out local, organic farmers, food co-ops, or community-supported agriculture (CSA) farms. These often have excellent selections and prices when it comes to organic food. Finally, we need to educate ourselves on why organic costs more. Contrary to some opinions, organic farmers are not trying to take advantage of you. It mainly comes down to subsidies, as well as supply and demand. There is also a higher risk of losing crops, and organic farming tends to be more labor and management intensive.

"If you think organic food is expensive, have you priced cancer lately?"

— Joel Salatin, author and founder of Polyface Farms

The other popular excuse some people use for not choosing organic is that they just don't trust that certified organic food is actually organic. Whether we feel jaded by the current political system or have heard stories of certifying agencies being influenced to say what corporations want them to say, this is definitely a very valid issue. So what is our solution? First, seek local farms. Get to know the farmers in your area, who is farming organically, and get to know them personally. Having a relationship with the person who provides your food is a sure way to be more empowered and feel more certain as to the quality of your food. Second, do some research about what organic certification actually means and how it is regulated. We tend to feel more confident about our choices when we are equipped with the right information. Ultimately, certification has gotten more controlled over the years, and not just anyone can claim to be an organic food provider. Today, there are several third-party or independent certifying agencies, and more steps are being taken to unify standards.

In this section, I also want to address an opposite-case scenario that can sometimes happen when people become too rigid about eating organic. Some are so fixated on making sure that everything is organic that they will not even touch fruits and vegetables if organics are not available. While I'll be the first to tell you to always choose organic over conventional, if it comes down to eating fruits and vegetables from non-organic sources or not eating them at all, your choice should always be to eat them. Despite their problems, the benefits of eating even non-organic fruits and vegetables outweigh not eating them at all. If your grocery store does not stock any organics and there is no other way for you to source them, eat whatever fruits and vegetables are available to you. On the other hand, if your grocery does not carry organic cherries but has other organic fruits, I would say pass on the cherries. Again, it comes down to being smart with our choices and any necessary tradeoffs. With respect to animal foods, I cannot say the same, simply because these are not necessary in our diet as fruits and vegetables are and typically carry more risks than benefits regardless of their production origin. If you are going to eat animal foods, only consider organic options.

Making Sense of What Organic Means

When it comes to eating organic, while we have come a long way in trusting what is and isn't really organic, there are still some who are skeptical or simply don't know what to expect. For starters, if a food item says "organic" on the label, it had to be certified by some third-party or governing body, such as the USDA, Ecocert, or QAI. The USDA National Organic Program (NOP) defines organic as follows:

> "Organic food is produced by farmers who emphasize the use of renewable resources and the conservation of soil and water to enhance environmental quality for future generations. Organic meat, poultry, eggs, and dairy products come from animals that are given no antibiotics or growth hormones. Organic food is produced without using most conventional pesticides; fertilizers made with synthetic ingredients or sewage sludge; bioengineering; or ionizing radiation. Before a product can be labeled organic, a Government-approved certifier inspects the farm where the food is grown to make sure the farmer is following all the rules necessary to meet USDA organic standards. Companies that handle or process organic food before it gets to your local supermarket or restaurant must be certified, too."

With the above definition in mind, yes, it takes some trust. However, as consumers like us become increasingly involved in how our food is grown, produced, and labeled, we are driving a positive change for our future. We demand accountability, and we are seeing more positive results when it comes to our food production. Again, the easiest and best way to truly eat organic is to find local farms, CSA programs, or markets and establish good relationships with the farmers who provide your food. Knowing how your food was grown, where it came from, and getting it at the peak of its freshness are all valuable for optimal health.

We must also remember not to get caught up in the "organic" label when it comes to processed food. Organic does not automatically mean healthy. First and foremost, it depends on the food. Our whole discussion here is based on buying organic whole, natural foods, whether from plants or animals. While we can easily find organic chips, cookies, and condiments today, these often defeat the very purpose of eating organic. If you are using them as transition items while you take steps on your optimal health journey and are sourcing out processed organic foods, they are definitely better than non-organic, but please don't stop there. The goal is whole, natural food that is also organic.

Practical Tips for Eating Organic

To finish this section, here are some tips for making the best choices when it comes to eating organic:

1. **Seek out local farmers, organic farms, or farmers' markets.**

2. **Consider joining a local, organic CSA program or food co-op.**

3. **When buying organic, make sure the label bears at least one third-party organic certification.**

4. **For financial savings and health benefits, buy organic produce that is in season and from local sources, as much as possible.**

5. **If eating animal products, always seek high-quality, free-range, pasture fed, organic sources.**

6. **If organic options are not available, still eat whole, natural plant foods. Non-organic fruits and vegetables are better than none.**

7. **Avoid high-risk GMO foods, unless they are organic, like corn, soy, canola, and sugar beets.**

8. **Do not be deceived by organic processed, refined, or otherwise unhealthy foods.**

PART 2
What to Eat for Optimal Health

"Health is a state of complete physical, mental, and social wellbeing, and not merely the absence of disease or infirmity."

— World Health Organization, 1948

CHAPTER 7
What Should We Really Eat?

Now that we have a good foundation of knowing how to eat, in this second part of the book, we will get more specific as to what to eat for optimal health and weight, healing, and prevention.

My personal journey of healthy eating has evolved over the years; it is now as easy and intuitive as I believe it was meant to be. This is not because I have a background in nutrition; my conventionally oriented biology degree certainly didn't help much in this area. Sure, it helped me understand the human body and the biochemical nature of some parts of nutrition, but it took several years and personal initiative for me to begin to connect the dots between how nutrition actually impacts our bodies. On my personal journey, I chose to go back to the basics, to relearn everything I thought I knew and approach healthy eating from nature's perspective. Everything changed, and a whole new world opened up to me when I decided to consciously examine what we are told to eat and the food choices I was making. I started to make connections between the foods we eat and the results within our bodies. I took into consideration what the majority of people are eating and the state of health they are exhibiting. I was not interested in becoming part of the disease statistics, and I learned there was a lot I could do to prevent that from happening. Perhaps I was fortunate: From an early age, I knew fast food and heavily refined foods do not belong in my body. However, there are so many foods and so many ingredients today, and education systems, even holistic ones, don't always teach us adequately about them. So I inquired, read, and learned, and I began to take personal accountability for my choices. I considered artificial colors and flavors, additives, synthetic nutrients, and modified ingredients, and I concluded that they do not belong in my body. I didn't need to wait for a doctor or government agency to tell me those things are bad for me. I knew for myself, and I know you do too. That innate knowing is within all of us.

People in our culture may eat this way, choosing taste, socially accepted norms, or convenience over health. Our parents may have eaten this way. Our friends and co-workers may still be. Nevertheless, optimal health is not about blindly following in the footsteps of others. Rather, it is about looking honestly at our food as the building blocks of our bodies, from which we derive the necessary fuel and nutrients. It is about seriously deciding what we feel is acceptable and beneficial to enter our system and what isn't. We don't think twice about putting the right fuel in our cars, yet when it comes to our bodies, for some reason we seem to think we can make exaggerated exceptions.

For many of us, the question of what to eat is no big deal until we become more conscious of the extreme impact our food has on our health and wellbeing. What we eat, what we put into our system, has the power to build, repair, and maintain the necessary balance. However, if we put junk in, we get junk in return. Our body and health are created from within, hence, the famous, "You are what you eat." If we are throwing in anything and everything that is currently allowed to be labeled as food in our society, we are treating our bodies more like a garbage can than anything of value. In fact, today, most garbage cans get better treatment; at least there, we take the time to carefully segregate the items according to where they actually belong. As for our bodies, many of us have yet to develop a deeper respect and appreciation for them, understanding that just because something is edible, that does not mean we should eat it. We need to be more discerning when it comes to what we allow to enter our bodies.

Today, we have more food choices than ever. On the other hand, though, we are privy to less real food than ever! This is what often leaves people confused, and they resort to items that are creating the weight and health problems no one wants to deal with. But while there may have been a shortage of information about the effects of fast and processed food on our bodies when it first came out, today we know with certainty that these foods will not lead to the weight and health we desire. There is also no question about the positive power of whole, natural plant foods. There is no study that will tell you not to eat fruits and vegetables and instead eat processed food. The ball is now in our court to take more accountability for our food choices. Deep down, I have to believe that we know that food for optimal health is meant to be natural, free of chemicals, wholesome, nutritious, and naturally great-tasting. We haven't lost our way completely. We have just become inundated with too many misleading choices that have been disguised as food. We have gotten caught up in the busyness of life, neglecting our most fundamental needs. We have allowed a veil to be placed over our eyes as to what real food and real health is supposed to be.

The choice to lift that veil and to see through the illusion is ours to make anytime, and until we do, our health and that of our families will continue to pay the price. Today, people suffer from more allergies and health conditions than ever before. Babies are being born with allergies and adverse conditions that were never before present. The top three diseases and killers in our society —heart disease, cancer, and diabetes—are preventable and lifestyle related. Our energy levels are so bad that most of us cannot start the day without external stimulants. We forgot how magnificent and powerful our bodies really are, and we think it is normal to regularly come down with infections. Headaches, indigestion, and sleep problems have become the norm for far too many. We need to snap out of this dream that has become a nightmare for so many of us. This is not how we were meant to live. We need to realize that none of this is "normal" or "natural"; it is a sign that our bodies are severely out of balance. We were constructed in such a brilliant, intelligent way. Our bodies are capable of magnificent things, one of which is knowing how to heal themselves and exist in perfect health. However, they are resilient only up to a point. When we push them too far, abuse them too much, or fail to give them the right support and resources, they let us know that something needs our attention. At that point, we can turn things around, but instead of doing so, most of us try to suppress the symptoms and carry on with our habits, as if nothing ever happened. Thus, our bodies are forced to communicate with us louder and louder, trying to get our attention in other ways, until something bigger comes along and we are overcome by some debilitating condition or disease.

No one wants to, needs to, or deserves to suffer. This is one of the main reasons why I decided to pursue the path of bringing as much awareness to this topic as possible. I have gained control over my own health and continue to be empowered by my daily supportive choices. I know firsthand that it is possible to feel great physically, mentally, and energetically every day, from morning to night! This is why I take what I eat very seriously. However, there is no deprivation, obsession, rigidity, or self-denial involved. Simply put, when you learn to look at all the so-called food out there through the lens of optimal health, you see just how inadequate it is when it comes to nourishing your body and how good it is at destroying your body and health. Although many choose to ignore facts and, even more precisely, ignore their body's desperate cries for help, it is generally hard to forget what you have learned. Once you become conscious of a new idea that resonates with you on some level, that idea will begin to grow. Before you know it, you'll feel a paradigm shift in your thinking, and you will start to see things from a new perspective. Once that happens, there is no going back. You will know, without a doubt, what is best for you, and no new diet, miracle supplement, or fancy advertising claim will shake that foundation.

What About "Everything in Moderation"?

This saying is one of my favorites, because it never ceases to amaze me what excuses we will use to justify poor habits or choices. Most people who spout off these words do so completely unconsciously, but it really is nothing more than a cop-out for not taking charge or personal accountability for our eating. It also doesn't help that this statement has become so culturally accepted that even the best of health professionals recite it without giving it a second thought. We are influenced by various addictions, traditions, peer pressure, ignorance, and convenience, all the while neglecting to understand that just because the human body can *tolerate* a substance without experiencing instant ill health or death, that does not mean it wants to or that we should expose ourselves to it. What is tolerable for us is simply not always good for us. I always say that if our bodies were see-through, so that we could see the stress and damage we cause with certain food items, we would make entirely different choices on the spot.

Another big reason why everything in moderation does not hold true is that there is no universal definition of what "moderation" means in regard to all the foods and beverages that are available to us. As we've seen with other words already, everyone has a different definition of *moderation*. What may qualify as moderation for one person is usually completely different for another. Does eating chocolate bars in moderation mean eating them once a day, once a week, or once a month? And what size of chocolate bar are we talking about? What if I am eating chocolate bars and French fries in moderation and washing them down with soda in moderation? Many people eat and drink junk daily but justify it because each item is only taken in their idea of moderation. In truth, there is no universal definition of moderation; there never was, and there never will be. It is senseless to think this overused statement will pave the way for optimal health and weight. In the end, we fail to realize just how much we are sabotaging our own health and wellbeing by using this ideology. Therefore, we can all do ourselves, our health, and our weight a huge favor right now by deciding that we will not use a moderation excuse to continue any of our destructive habits. If we are okay with everything in moderation, we also have to be prepared to experience health and weight problems in moderation.

Isn't the Food Guide or Pyramid Enough?

On the journey of becoming more mindful about our food choices, the first place many people turn is to a resource that was developed to help us know what to eat. In the United States, this is called the Food Pyramid; in Canada, it is known as the Food Guide. While both have undergone some serious upgrades in the past few years, they still fall short in many areas when it comes to helping people understand what food to eat and how much of it.

For starters, these are misleading, suggesting that eating from the four major food groups will ensure good health. Millions of optimally healthy people never eat dairy and/or meat. Furthermore, until not that long ago, these resources included many foods that are far from healthy. For years, both suggested grains as the main food source, with the Canadian Food Guide recommending five to twelve servings a day! Out of those pictured, almost all were refined, white products. Second, the guides do not cover all foods, so this leaves people guessing and coming to their own conclusions. As mentioned, these resources have already been revised several times because they simply do not serve the general public well. Most people still have a hard time understanding serving sizes and ideal food choices. The guides do not address food quality or preparation either.

So, while both offer a basic foundation as to where we should begin, these resources should be viewed as guides for attaining average health at best. If we want optimal health, we need to take things into our own hands.

The Path of Knowing What to Eat

The key to successful healthy eating and the easiest way to know what to eat is not to list all the things that don't belong in our bodies. Frankly, there are far too many to list. Rather, we should focus on what does belong on our menus. We also shouldn't attempt to focus on the things we cannot have, as this will only make us want them more. In essence, you can have anything you want, but the question is what will you want once you align with your health and weight priorities. Allow your natural knowing to guide you. Also, take things step by step, at your own pace, progressing as you feel ready. Focus on the right stuff and let the wrong stuff fall away on its own. This is what I recommend for everyone, whether you are interested in changing your dietary habits, improving your health, or losing weight. Start by incorporating more healthy choices into each day. Slowly but surely, as you learn more about the value of each natural, wholesome food choice and see and feel the results in your wellbeing, you will naturally continue to gravitate toward them, losing your interest and taste for the fake or unhealthy food.

Here is a simple summary of what to eat for optimal health:

1. **Fruits and Vegetables**
2. **Beans and Legumes**
3. **Whole, Unprocessed Grains**
4. **Nuts and Seeds**
5. **Minimal Animal Products**
6. **Water**
7. **Other Foods** (mushrooms, herbs, etc.)

Note: Specific foods within the groups will be categorized based on their most common uses. Some may, thus, overlap in groups or categories to diversify their usage.

This list is short, yet it offers endless and exciting combinations. Short is also good because it is meant to be simple and intuitive. Healthy eating is not complicated; it is all about real food of the right type. Once you know what to eat, simply apply how to it eat, focusing on its natural, raw, and organic forms. By eating plant-based, with a focus on fruits, vegetables, and leafy greens, you will naturally be eating in alignment with the acid-alkaline balance as well. It all fits synchronistically, and it all works synergistically!

Eating the above foods in their most wholesome forms will mimic what the human body is used to from an evolutionary perspective, with beneficial adaptations for our times. To date, this has been shown to be the most optimal nourishment for our health, weight, and overall wellbeing. We did not evolve on mac and cheese, marshmallows, or hotdogs. Our bodies need real food and real nutrients. In the next seven chapters, we will address the above list in more detail, to better understand the importance and value of each item and how to best work with them in your diet.

CHAPTER 8
Fruits & Vegetables

The value and importance of fruits and vegetables has been presented many times in the first part of this book. In this chapter, we will take a closer look at them and share some practical ways to incorporate them into our diets.

High Nutrients, Low Calories

Fruits and vegetables contain the highest concentrations of vitamins, minerals, antioxidants, and phytonutrients. They are nutritional powerhouses and offer all this to us for a fraction of the calories, as compared to other foods.

Fruits are higher in calories, as compared to vegetables, so they can be fantastic, quick energy sources. They are extremely easy to digest and taste really good too!

Vegetables are lower in calories and while they are mostly devoid of simple sugars, they still taste great especially after our taste buds detox from all the fake foods. Veggies make great snacks, as well as diverse meal combinations.

Fiber

Fruits and vegetables are excellent sources of fiber. When people experience any kind of digestive upset, such as constipation, all too often, they run to the drugstore for fiber pills and powders. In most cases, all it would take is a trip to the produce section, as fruits and vegetables offer excellent support for healthy, regular elimination.

An interesting point to make here is that sometimes, due to various influences, some of us are reluctant to eat fruit, too many fruits, or fruits of a certain kind, due to their sugar content. What we need to realize, however, is that the sugar in fruits is wholesome, bound to various beneficial nutrients. With the help of its inherent fiber, it does not carry the same blood-glucose-spiking effect as cookies and soda and even most refined, white flour foods. It never ceases to amaze me that some try to pick apart real, natural plant food but choose to overlook so many processed and animal foods that are the *real* problem. Whole-food, plant-based physicians who specialize in lifestyle disease reversal and healing, like Drs. Joel Fuhrman or Gabriel Cousens, successfully help people lose weight and even reverse diabetes while including fruit as a regular part or even large part of the diet.

Macronutrients

Both fruits and vegetables offer healthy sources of carbohydrates and are naturally very low in fat. The main exception being the avocado that contains a myriad of healthy fats. Yes, fruits and vegetables contain protein; this is an idea many of us have yet to get used to. In fact, vegetables, especially those from the cruciferous family, as well as leafy greens, exhibit excellent protein profiles. Spinach, for example, is one of the highest-protein plant foods, with about 50 percent of its calories coming from protein.

Micronutrients

When it comes to micronutrients, our vitamins and minerals, both fruits and vegetables are rich sources of nearly all of them. This is why I mentioned in Chapter 3 that it is not a good idea to associate specific fruits and vegetables with specific vitamins or minerals. No food is a single nutrient. To think of them as such limits their immense potential and is partly to blame for our unfounded nutritional fears. When we eat an abundant and varied diet based on fruits and vegetables, we consume a diet rich in vitamins and minerals, all in their most natural form.

The exceptions to the above statements, as also shared in Chapter 3, include Vitamins D and B12. As far as we know at this time, no fruit or vegetable contains Vitamin D, which is technically more of a hormone than a nutrient. Hence, we must source this important compound elsewhere. Sun exposure on our skin is the best and most natural method, when done mindfully. Vitamin

B12 is synthesized by certain bacteria in our environment. Therefore, fruits and vegetables can contain it extrinsically, as residual from manure or bacterial contamination. Levels of B12 on fruits and vegetables depend on the soil they are grown in and how vigorously and thoroughly they are washed; frankly, given our conventional produce and sanitary practices, modern fruits and vegetables cannot be construed as a reliable source of B12.[1] Our ancestors and some cultures who continue to farm and live naturally would have access to B12 from their plants, but we cannot count on this given our modern society. Vitamin B12-like compounds, analogues, have been found in certain plant foods, but these do not appear to satisfy our B12 needs and may even hinder our B12 absorption.[2] Although technically not vegetables or even plants, mushrooms have been more prominently considered as reliable sources of Vitamin D and B12, and we will talk about them in Chapter 14.

Healing & Prevention

Countless research over the decades has shown positive correlations between fruits and vegetables and our health, especially for healing and prevention. While each fruit and vegetable is beneficial to us, there is a catch: For the most significant benefits, they must be consumed in significant amounts. It is great to eat an apple or banana and some lettuce leaves and tomato slices each day, but this is merely the tip of the iceberg. As I have been sharing with you throughout this book, these foods will do wonders for us in terms of weight loss, healing, and reversal of disease, as well as prevention against future states of disease, but they must be the main part of our diet, included in every meal rather than just an occasional side dish. If we look within, beyond the fake foods and corporately-driven cultural trends, we know innately that these are the two food types around which our diets should revolve.

What makes fruits and veggies so powerful at healing, prevention, and ensuring optimal health is that they are ideally suited to aid our body and health, offering us top sources of nutrition for the present and advantages for the future. In fact, their nutrient amounts appear to be perfectly suited for the needs of the human body. They are highly anti-inflammatory, alkalizing, energizing, cleansing, and detoxifying. They offer incredible antioxidant activity and other countless benefits, thanks to their unique phytonutrients. Diets based on large quantities of fresh fruits and vegetables have been found to strongly support and enhance the immune system and promote ideal weight, overall good health, and longevity. They are protective against all cancers, heart disease, and diabetes. Likewise, they are used in the healing and reversal of these conditions, as well as many others. They are also easily enjoyed in their most natural, raw form, making fruits and vegetables true all-stars to benefit from in our daily diet.

Fruit & Vegetable Choices for You

What fruits and vegetables do you eat daily? If you are like most, you have a common handful of usual choices, but there are thousands of them out there to choose from! While it is always best to eat organic and local produce, as discussed previously, we can take advantage of many non-local fruits and vegetables today as well. Our grocery stores may not be able to supply them all, but few of us even eat a quarter of those that are stocked in the produce department.

Below are some fruit and vegetables that are commonly found in most North American grocery stores, farmers' markets, and personal gardens. Skim the list for those you've never heard of or tried, and consider putting them in your shopping basket next time. Make it a point to diversify your choices in these two areas. You can also make it a fun challenge to try at least one of every type of fruit and vegetable your grocery store carries. Apart from the different types in each group, there are many different varieties of each type, too, depending upon where you live. Also, remember that while organic options are best, make a point of eating a large portion of vegetables and fruits, even if you cannot find the organic varieties. Thorough washing (and peeling when appropriate and necessary) can help decrease the pesticide load of non-organic varieties.

Fruits

Berry Fruits: Strawberry, Raspberry, Blueberry, Blackberry, Gooseberry, Cranberry, Acai Berry, Goji Berry, Bilberry, Winterberry, Ligonberry

Stone Fruits: Apricot, Cherry, Peach, Plum, Nectarine

Citrus Fruits: Tangerine, Mandarine, Clementine, Orange, Lemon, Lime, Grapefruit, Pomelo

Tropical Fruits: Pineapple, Banana, Mango, Papaya, Coconut, Guava, Passion Fruit, Dragon Fruit

Melon Fruits: Honeydew, Cantaloupe, Watermelon, Santa Claus Melon, Canary Melon

Other Fruits: Apple, Pear, Kiwi, Pomegranate, Currants, Grapes, Fuyu Persimmon, Fig, Date, Lychee, Pawpaw, Breadfruit, Cactus Pear

Vegetables

Fruit Vegetables: Tomato, Avocado, Cucumber, Eggplant, Okra, Olives, Bell Pepper, Zucchini, Pumpkin, Butternut Squash, Buttercup Squash, Spaghetti Squash, Acorn Squash

Bulb Vegetables: Onions, Garlic, Chives, Leeks, Scallions, Shallots

Leaf Vegetables: Romaine Lettuce, Green or Red Leaf Lettuce, Boston Lettuce, Spinach, Arugula, Brussels Sprouts, Cabbage, Collard Greens, Kale, Swiss Chard, Watercress, Dandelion, Nettles, Endive, Purslane, Radicchio, Savoy, Bok Choy, Sorrel, Mustard Greens

Root Vegetables: Beets, Carrots, Celeriac, Parsnips, Radish, Rutabaga, Turnips

Inflorescence Vegetables: Artichokes, Broccoli, Cauliflower

Stalk Vegetables: Asparagus, Bamboo, Celery, Rhubarb, Fiddlehead, Fennel, Kohlrabi

Tuber Vegetables: Potato, Sweet Potato, Yam, Cassava, Taro, Jerusalem Artichoke, Jicama

Seed/Pod Vegetables: Green Beans, Yellow Beans, Green Peas, Snow Peas, Edamame, Corn

Sea Vegetables: Arame, Dulse, Kombu, Nori, Sea Palm, Wakame

Practical Tips for Eating Fruits & Vegetables

To finish this section, here are some tips for making the most of fruits and vegetables in your diet:

1. **Eat more vegetables than fruits each day.** Every meal should be vegetable-based, and snacks can be fruit-based. For optimal digestion it is best to eat fruits on their own or with water-rich vegetables including leafy greens and not eat them directly after main meals due to their rapid digestion.

2. **From the vegetable group, focus most on leafy greens and the cruciferous family of vegetables.** Leafy greens include: kale, collard greens, spinach, or lettuces and are excellent for use raw, in daily whole-meal green smoothies and salads. Cruciferous vegetables include: broccoli, cauliflower, cabbage, or brussel sprouts, and are excellent steamed and in daily veggie-based main dishes. (Some overlap both groups.)

3. **Eat according to what is in season.** Apply this tip to both fruits and vegetables, but especially fruits, enjoying a wide variety of seasonal varieties. If you live in North America, here are some general seasonal guidelines: Berries should be our main late spring through summer choices; stone fruits, apples, and pears should be our main late summer through fall choices; and citrus and tropical fruits should be our main winter to early spring choices.

4. **Eat all colors of fruits and vegetables.** You know you are on the right track when your meals are full of vibrant, natural colors. Whether it is a bright green whole-meal breakfast smoothie, a rainbow colored whole-meal lunch salad, a dark purple afternoon snack based on berries, or a cream-colored dinner dish based on potatoes and cauliflower, enjoy the visually appealing creations and their accompanying flavor sensations!

5. **Eat organic as much as possible.**

6. **Eat raw as much as possible.** Recall that this can easily include steamed and lightly cooked options.

7. **Don't forget about the sea vegetables.** Nori, dulse, and wakame are some of the healthiest, most nutrient-rich plant foods. We will discuss these in Chapter 14.

8. **Avoid canned fruit, fruit cups, and commercial fruit juices.** Fruits from cans are normally heat treated, destroying most of their valuable nutrients. Since they are acidic prior to digestion, this does not make for a healthy reaction with the can either. Most food cans contain liners, which commonly include a toxic, hormone-disrupting chemical called BPA. As for fruit cups and fruit juices, these normally contain added sugars, have been heat treated (pasteurized), and in the case of juices are missing the valuable fiber, while being a source of empty liquid calories. To add to this, most of these products are so artificially produced that they should not be counted in any way as fruit servings or optimally healthy choices. Think fresh, raw, and wholesome!

9. **Avoid canned vegetables and commercial vegetable juices.** One look at canned vegetables, and the color and texture should give you some clue as to the lack of nutritional quality. Like canned fruit, they are high-heat treated and sit in cans for months before we consume them. Your number-one choice should always be real, whole, and fresh. If you cannot go that route, frozen is second best. Commercial vegetable juices are heavily processed, normally high in sodium and typically contain added sugars, colors, flavors, and preservatives. Also, they typically come in plastic bottles or aluminum-lined cartons, neither of which are good for optimal health.

10. **Fruit and vegetable meal ideas:** Fruits and vegetables can make various smoothies, salads, soups, stews, stir-fries, sauces, spreads, bars, raw and frozen desserts, snacks, shakes, and more! We will cover some specific and practical meal examples in Chapter 15.

CHAPTER 9
Beans & Legumes

Beans and legumes are all too often neglected by most people as part of a regular diet for a variety of reasons. Some of us don't know what to do with them. Some think they are a hassle to work unless they are canned, and many don't want to bother with their preparation. Some are simply afraid of the possible digestive consequences. Still others just don't give them enough thought to realize how amazing they are from a nutritional, health, satiety, and economical perspective. A diet devoid of beans and legumes is missing out on a vital, nutrient-rich, inexpensive, and highly versatile food source. Let's take a closer look at these nutritional powerhouses.

Nutrients & Calories

Like fruits and vegetables, beans and legumes contain high concentrations of vitamins, minerals, antioxidants, and phytonutrients. They are also low in calories and rich in nutrients, making them a very health- and weight-friendly food source.

Fiber

One of their greatest assets and claims to fame is their fiber content. Beans and legumes contain both soluble and insoluble fiber, so they are highly valuable for optimal digestion, especially a healthy colon and regular elimination. They also assist in optimal cholesterol regulation, blood glucose regulation, blood pressure regulation, detoxification, and weight maintenance.

Macronutrients

Beans and legumes are outstanding sources of protein. Being a plant food, beans and legumes provide us with both an optimal quantity and quality of protein for the human body. They are a source of healthy, complex carbohydrates, with virtually no sugar or fat. Also, like all plant foods, they are cholesterol-free.

Micronutrients

Like fruits and vegetables, beans and legumes are a source of almost every vitamin and mineral, except for Vitamins B12 and D. They are some of the highest sources of vital minerals like iron, zinc, magnesium, potassium, and calcium. Also like fruits and vegetables, each bean variety has its own particular strengths in its micronutrient profile. Therefore, a diet that regularly includes a wide variety of different beans is best to maximize the various health, healing, and prevention benefits they offer. Soaked and/or sprouted beans are typically higher in many micronutrients.

Healing & Prevention

Due to their amazing fiber and nutrient density, beans and legumes provide healing and prevention for many conditions including: cancers (especially colon), heart disease, hypertension, Type 2 diabetes and blood sugar regulation, irritable bowel syndrome, osteoporosis, and weight gain. They enhance overall good health and are an outstanding part of an optimally healthy diet.

Bean & Legume Choices for You

Similarly to fruits and vegetables, most people are only familiar with a small variety of beans. The average grocery store carries at least a dozen different kinds in the dry section and several others in the fresh and frozen sections. Some fresh beans are best enjoyed raw, but most beans and legumes are best consumed cooked or sprouted. Dry beans are extremely versatile, and almost all cook in a similar fashion. Typically, most dry beans and some lentils, should be soaked in ample water before cooking. Soaking times will vary depending on the type of bean or legume, but commonly range from eight to twenty-four hours. For the sake of simplicity, soak beans overnight to cook the following day. When you are ready to cook, drain the water they have been soaked in, rinse well, cover with ample fresh water, and bring to a boil; reduce the heat to simmer and continue cooking on low heat. Depending on the bean type, they will take about thirty to sixty minutes to cook on low heat, after having been properly soaked; some lentils will take as little as ten minutes to cook even without soaking. To keep your dry beans or legumes raw, you can soak and sprout them. Sprouting times vary between varieties, but it typically takes two to four days. Enjoy exploring the many varieties and forms available.

Different varieties include:

- Adzuki Beans (also known as Field Peas or Red Oriental Beans)
- Anasazi Beans (also known as Jacob's Cattle Beans)
- Black Beans (also known as Turtle Beans)
- Black-Eyed Peas (also known as Cowpeas)
- Cranberry Beans
- Edamame (also known as Green Soybeans)
- Fava Beans (also known as Broad or Horse Beans)
- Garbanzo Beans (also known as Chickpeas or Ceci Beans)
- Garden Peas
- Great Northern Beans
- Green Beans (also known as Snap or String Beans)
- Kidney Beans
- Lentils (various types)
- Lima Beans (also known as Butter or Madagascar Beans)
- Lupine Beans
- Mung Beans
- Navy Beans
- Pigeon Peas
- Pinto Beans
- Romano Beans (also known as Roman or Borlotti beans)
- Snow Peas (also known as Chinese Pea Pods)
- Sugar Snap Peas
- Soybeans (also known as Soynuts)

- Sweet Peas
- White Beans
- Yellow Split Peas
- Yellow Wax Beans (also known as Snap or String Beans)

Practical Tips for Eating Beans & Legumes

To finish this section, here are some tips for making the most of beans and legumes in your diet:

1. **Eat a wide variety of beans and legumes regularly.** Refer to the list in the previous section for new ideas. Enjoy fresh beans and legumes seasonally and frozen ones when fresh are not available or in season. Aim to include at least one bean or legume serving daily.

2. **Eat dry beans, not canned.** As already discussed, canned foods are not optimal for our health. If you need to rely on them, they should be the exception rather than the rule. Dry beans have an excellent shelf life, are economical, and can be sprouted or cooked when desired. To reduce cooking time and improve nutrition, soak beans in ample water overnight.

3. **At first, include beans and legumes in small portions in your meals to allow your intestines to adjust.** Excessive bloating or gas after eating beans can be due to numerous factors, such as improper enzyme function, improper food combining, improper gut microflora due to processed-food diets or antibiotic use, improper bean preparation, and general poor intestinal health. Incorporate beans slowly into your diet if you are not used to them; this will allow your intestines and digestive system to adjust accordingly. When we clean up our diet, we clean up our intestines, and this improves the digestion of all foods. Longer soaking times also decrease the potential of any digestive disturbances. It is completely possible to enjoy beans and legumes regularly without any digestive disturbances.

4. **Get creative with your bean and legume meal ideas.** Beans and legumes can be used in numerous salads, soups, stews, stir-fries, wraps, veggie burger patties, dips, sauces, spreads, and purées; or easily added as a side dish to almost any meal.

CHAPTER 10
Whole, Unprocessed Grains

Grains have had quite an eventful ride as part of our food supply. For thousands of years, specifically since their inclusion as common agricultural food staples some 10,000 years ago, we have used them in their crude form. Then, during the past 200 years or so, since the inception of large grain mills (some research indicates even earlier), we began refining grains, stripping them of their most nutritionally dense parts and even subjecting them to chemicals. Industrialized societies began to prize a refined, white product, unaware of how destructive such processing is for our health. It was considered a positive advancement for storage, shipping, and overall appeal. It wasn't until the early 1900s, when we learned about the different vitamins, minerals, and amino acids, that we began to realize that the parts we were so haphazardly stripping away were the most nutritious. Even then, however, instead of leaving grains whole, we tackled the problem by enriching white flour with synthetic nutrients, since it was rather nutritionally worthless on its own. It took us a while, but we finally learned conclusively that grains are healthiest in their whole form; some records indicate that ancient cultures knew this much earlier. Products made from white, refined flour lead to a whole slew of weight and disease problems. Upon realizing the health implications related to refined grain products, our transition into the twenty-first century paved the way for a movement back to using grains in their whole form.

The destructive qualities of refined grains are not only related to what they lost but also to what they took on during their refining and processing. It is great that we are now experiencing a resurgence of whole grain popularity, but if these grains are part of processed foods, it simply isn't enough for optimal health and weight. Knowing what we know today when it comes to the health problems associated with refined grains, it is unfortunate that the vast majority of us are not doing more to change our processed grain habits. Not only do white flour products necessitate the removal of the healthiest grain components, like the bran and germ, but they also undergo various bleaching and chemical treatments. Whether white or brown (whole), flour-based products do not bode well for our health and weight.

It is nice to see "whole grain" on the labels of many processed foods today, but we must realize that it is one thing to eat a whole grain where we actually see the grain in its natural, whole form and quite another to eat a processed product made from whole grains. These are certainly not equal; neither in their nutrition nor effects on our health. This is why when I refer to whole grains, I specify them as unprocessed; this makes a huge difference in our health in terms of the nutritional quality of the food. Unlike whole, actual grains, flour (white or whole), due to its large surface area, is digested more like a simple sugar than a complex carbohydrate. Eating products made from flour results in more blood-glucose irregularities, putting us at risk for developing Type 2 diabetes and also gaining weight. Secondly, if we examine the average bread-like product in our stores or bakeries, even those that proudly display "whole grain" on their labels, refined flower (white, enriched, or unbleached) will almost always be found on the ingredient list as well, amidst other undesirable ingredients like sugars, hydrogenated vegetable oils, modified food ingredients, preservatives, and so on.

Another problem when it comes to grains, as mentioned in Chapter 3, is that we rely on them too heavily as part of our daily meals. Many people start the day off with boxed cereals, bagels, or muffins, have a sandwich or pita for lunch, and often finish the day with pasta or pizza for dinner. Bread and bread-like products, cakes, cookies, crackers, boxed cereals, and pastas are generally copiously eaten by the average person in our society. They are also the most commonly used foods to appease children who are picky eaters. These are not nutritionally sound products. They are great at filling us up, providing us with ample calories, and making meal times relatively easy and fast, but they do not provide our bodies with what they really need or serve our health well in any way. From Chapter 4, you hopefully recall the importance of the acid-alkaline balance. At their best, grains are usually mildly acid-forming; at their worst, they are very acid-forming. This is another important reason to only use them in their whole, unprocessed forms, and consume alongside other wholesome ingredients.

There are so many different grains out there, yet our society seems to be greatly intent on exploiting just one: wheat. According to *World's Healthiest Foods*, wheat is the most important cereal crop in the world. Whenever a crop is so heavily capitalized and depended on, it tends to be quite problematic, due to the various modifications, hybridizations, and chemical treatments it undergoes to ensure a profitable yield. Each day, more people learn that they have a sensitivity or intolerance to wheat or even all *gluten*, a protein component found in many grains, especially in modern wheat. Speaking of gluten, we are currently experiencing a gluten-free wave in our society, with many people opting for this dietary route even when they do not need to. Gluten though is not our main problem. Rather, it is primarily refined grains and modern wheat. If we make the switch from processed wheat products to processed gluten-free products, we may be avoiding wheat and gluten but we are still subjecting ourselves to all sorts of undesirable, acid-forming ingredients. Yes, gluten-free may be a nice or necessary way to go, but it should still be done with a reliance on real, whole foods for optimal health, weight, healing, and prevention. In fact, if you follow the guidelines provided in this book, your diet will naturally be very low in gluten, if not entirely gluten-free. Some of the best grain foods are seed grains like quinoa, millet, amaranth, and buckwheat, which are not true grains and naturally gluten-free. Therefore, make use of the many other grains out there in your culinary endeavors, especially natural gluten-free options like the ones mentioned above. When it comes to wheat, there are many varieties so opt for organic wheat or spelt and Kamut (a type of Khorasan wheat), which are ancient species of wheat and more wholesome and healthful than modern, conventional wheat. Be sure to read all food ingredient labels as well. Today, numerous products add extra gluten, and this can aggravate your intestinal and overall health.

Given all this, you may be wondering if grains are valuable for us at all. The answer is simple: Most definitely! We will explore their health benefits below. Natural, unrefined, whole grains can be an excellent and very healthy part of our diet. It all depends on the type, quantity, and quality. As mentioned previously, the healthiest way to consume grains, aside from whole, natural, and organic, is soaked, sprouted, or fermented. This decreases their nutritional inhibitors while increasing their nutritional value and ease of digestibility.

Nutrients & Calories

Whole, unprocessed grains tend to be comparable in calories to beans and legumes. They provide an outstanding source of energy, with nutritionally dense calories. We must remember that the body's optimal fuel is glucose, and we can supply it in the healthiest way via fruits and foods that are naturally rich in complex carbohydrates, such as beans and grains. Being a plant food, grains are also a good source of vitamins, minerals, antioxidants, and phytonutrients. According to *World's Healthiest Foods*, whole grains are important dietary sources of water-soluble, fat-soluble, and insoluble antioxidants. These multifunctional antioxidants are available along the digestive tract, offering immediate and long-term benefits, and research now indicates that the amount and activity of antioxidants in whole grains has been vastly underestimated in the past.[1]

Fiber

Grains left in their whole, unprocessed form retain their most valuable qualities: micronutrients and fiber. By eating white breads, pastas, and similar products, we are missing out on the best part of the food, consuming many things we shouldn't in the process. Similarly the fiber value of all flour, whether from whole or refined grains, is also not quite the same as eating actual whole grains. Whole, unprocessed grains are rich sources of fiber, and this offers positive effects for our digestive, cholesterol, blood-glucose, and cardiovascular health. As discussed in our previous chapters, fiber offers excellent protective properties against our common chronic diseases.

Macronutrients

Whole, unprocessed grains are an excellent source of healthy, complex carbohydrates. As these are digested, they provide a steady release of glucose, the body's optimal fuel. They are also a great source of protein and some healthy fat.

Micronutrients

Like beans and legumes, grains are an especially rich source of most minerals and B vitamins. Similar to our previous plant foods, grains cannot be depended on for Vitamins B12 or D. Soaked, sprouted, or fermented grains are typically higher in micronutrients.

Healing & Prevention

Whole, unprocessed grains have a favorable nutrient and fiber profile. When eaten in balanced portions, along with fruits, vegetables, beans, and legumes, they can serve as an optimally healthy food. Their healing and prevention properties have been most notably linked to all sorts of benefits and protection for our cardiovascular system, like supporting healthy blood pressure and preventing heart attacks and strokes. Thanks to their valuable antioxidants and phytonutrients, they offer many benefits for our immune system and cancer protection, especially of the breast or colon. Whole, unprocessed grains also lower the risk of Type 2 diabetes, as they do not spike blood-glucose levels unnaturally. They support optimal brain function, providing us with the necessary energy for our cognitive needs, and offer many optimal health and longevity benefits.

Whole Grain Choices for You

As with other foods in the plant kingdom, we have an incredible and abundant variety of grains to choose from. I encourage you to explore all the options, significantly reducing your reliance on conventional wheat. The same thing goes for corn, which should only be consumed in its organic, fresh form, not in its many processed forms or in other processed foods. We get the most nutrition, healing, and prevention benefits when we diversify our food choices and eat a wide array of foods rather than eating the same things regularly. Opt for organic, wholesome grain options, as well as soaked, sprouted, or fermented grain foods.

Here are some grain options for you to include in your diet. I have also mentioned which are gluten-free:

- Amaranth (gluten-free)
- Barley
- Bran of Various Grains (some gluten-free)
- Brown Rice (numerous varieties, gluten-free)
- Buckwheat (gluten-free)
- Bulgur
- Corn (gluten-free)
- Freekeh
- Indian Ricegrass (gluten-free)
- Kamut
- Millet (gluten-free)
- Oats (gluten-free)*
- Quinoa (gluten-free)
- Rye
- Sorghum (gluten-free)
- Spelt
- Teff (gluten-free)
- Wild Rice (gluten-free)

*Oats are commonly prone to gluten contamination. If you require a strictly gluten-free product, source certified gluten-free oats.

Practical Tips for Eating Grains

To finish this section, here are some tips for making the most of grains:

1. **Consume whole, unprocessed grains in their most natural form.** Any grains you choose to include in your regular diet should be whole and unprocessed. Refer to the list in the previous section for new ideas.

2. **Buy dry, natural grains, and cook them yourself.** Grains can be soaked to reduce cooking time and enhance their nutrient and digestibility profiles. Depending on the grain, cooking time varies from about two minutes (oat bran) to forty-five minutes (brown rice). An excellent company that

provides a wide variety of whole, unprocessed grains, including many organic options is Bob's Red Mill (widely available in U.S. and Canada).

3. **Avoid boxed cereals.** Although some companies are trying to create so-called healthier boxed cereals based on real, whole and minimally processed grains and dried fruits, when you examine the ingredients list, you will find that most still include things that are not optimal for our health, including too many simple, isolated sugars.

4. **Make grains a part of some meals but not the main part of any meal.** If you choose to start your day with a bowl of steel-cut oats, for example, the optimal thing to do would be to make sure that the rest of your meals are rich with leafy greens and vegetables. Otherwise, add only about half a cup to a cup of cooked grain to one or two of your main vegetable-based meals. Note that these are very broad and general guidelines; you should work with them in accordance with your age, health, and weight, bearing your physical activity level in mind.

5. **Avoid commercial cookies, crackers, granola bars, bagels, etc.** These are all heavily processed foods. It is tempting to eat them often, as they make easy snacks or meals, but they are in no way optimally healthy choices. They are loaded with sugar, in addition to many other undesirable ingredients, and act like sugar upon their digestion. The consumption of these products readily leads to weight gain, chronic acidosis, blood-glucose spikes, and all sorts of other health problems. It is, however, possible to make many wholesome, predominantly grainless, and even raw cookies, crackers, or granola bars at home in minutes. These can healthfully replace their processed counterparts.

6. **If eating bread, choose high-quality, pure, whole-grain breads, such as Ezekiel or sourdough, and consume them infrequently.** Please note that not all Ezekiel and sourdough breads are guaranteed to be optimally healthy. Read all ingredients to make sure your choice of bread only contains whole grains, preferably sprouted, and no refined flour, sugars, hydrogenated fats, or preservatives. Two excellent companies that make high-quality, flourless, sprouted grain breads are Food for Life and Manna Bread; their products can be easily found in the U.S. and Canada, typically in the frozen section,

as the breads are completely natural. Food for Life also offers optimally healthy Ezekiel wraps, which have outstanding ingredients and can be used for quick, wholesome veggie wraps.

7. **Avoid commercial baked goods and regular home baking.** Commercial baked goods and most home-baked goods are typically based on some of the unhealthiest fats and carbohydrates, like refined oils, flours, sugars, or other sweeteners, as well as a slew of additives, modified ingredients, and preservatives. The presence of high and prolonged heat, as well as the acid-forming effect, further substantiates why these should be avoided and not included in your diet for healing and prevention. Instead, opt for the numerous healthy options of raw, wholesome, and plant-based desserts that can be made without the need to completely destroy our food or add to it unfavorable ingredients.

8. **Get creative with your grain meal ideas.** Whole, unprocessed grains can be used as a side to various meals, including breakfast, lunch or dinner.

CHAPTER 11
Nuts & Seeds

Until recently, nuts and seeds have commonly been overlooked as part of a regular diet and used only sporadically as holiday or special event treats. Many people stay away from them in fear of their high-fat profiles. On the contrary, nuts and seeds offer superior nutrition and health benefits when in their whole, raw forms, so they should be part of our regular diet. Like so many other good-for-us, natural foods, they simply need to be enjoyed in a smart way.

When it comes to their fat content, while it is true that they are high in fat, we have to remember that fat is an essential nutrient, one our bodies need. There are different types of fats, and nuts and seeds are packed with a variety of healthy ones, including some omega-3 fatty acids. Like the sugar in fruits, there is no need to fear and avoid the fat in nuts. What we should be concerned about and avoid are the unhealthy sugars and fats that come with processed and junk foods. When incorporated as part of a healthy, plant-based diet, both nuts and seeds offer many health benefits, and they should actually be eaten for the very reason people avoid them: their fat content. With the exception of avocados, most fruits, vegetables, beans, legumes, and grains are naturally very low in fat. This is why nuts and seeds can be a complement, providing us with high-quality fats we may not get from other sources.

Nuts, which biologically are seeds as well, are inherently programmed to produce a new fruiting plant of its kind, and are thus packed with highly valuable nutrients to make that happen. This also applies to grains and beans; in essence, these are also a type of seed. Of course, not all seeds carry the same nutrient profiles. Some excel in carbohydrates, some in protein, and others in fat. When we consume these foods, specifically in their most natural and wholesome forms, we get the best of all and easily meet our nutritional requirements.

Another interesting fact is that when we are in tune with our bodies and they are working in a relatively balanced fashion, it is rare for us to overeat natural, raw nuts and seeds. They are a source of extremely dense energy, and our system has its own regulatory way of telling us when we have had enough; it usually doesn't take many nuts or seeds before we get to that point. It is most common for people to overindulge in these foods when they are heavily processed, roasted and covered in salt, sugar, and/or other flavored substances. The addictive nature of those substances is what is primarily responsible for causing us to eat the nuts or seeds uncontrollably. A general, average quantity of natural, raw nuts or seeds is about one-quarter cup or one small handful per serving, with about one to two servings per day. This will of course vary based on your personal health, age, and lifestyle needs and even the seasons; our bodies typically want lighter meals during the warmer months and more dense meals during the colder months.

Nutrients & Calories

As mentioned already, nuts and seeds are packed with nutrients. Like all plant foods, these include valuable minerals, vitamins, antioxidants, and phytonutrients. Unlike all other plant foods, though, nuts and seeds are very high in calories. This can work for or against us, depending on how and when we use them. They can be an excellent and very rich source of energy and healthy fats for those partaking in a whole-food, plant-based diet, considering that other whole plant foods are so naturally low in calories and fat. If you are still growing and/or are very active, you can eat more nuts and seeds daily; on the other hand, if you are trying to lose weight, you should aim to eat less nuts and seeds daily.

Fiber

Like all plant foods, nuts and seeds are a great source of fiber. As we previously discussed, high-fiber diets are associated with many benefits. These include: supporting our digestive health, regulating bowel movements, blood sugar and cholesterol, supporting healthy weight and weight-loss, and being protective against cancer, heart disease and Type 2 diabetes.

Macronutrients

Nuts and seeds primarily supply us with healthy fats. They are a great source of high-quality protein and healthy carbohydrates. They are rich in various fatty acids, mostly unsaturated, but they also contain some healthy saturated fatty acids, omega-6 fatty acids, and valuable omega-3 fatty acids.

Aside from being nutritional all-stars, hemp, flax, and chia seeds specifically provide nearly perfect omega-3-to-omega-6 ratios. In fact, flax and chia seeds are uniquely valuable foods, in that they offer more omega-3 than omega-6 fatty acids. Most foods, especially processed foods, animal foods, and refined oils, provide too much omega-6 and not enough omega-3, if any; this has been linked to our high levels of inflammation and chronic disease. We will explore these fats and the significance of this ratio further in Chapter 16. Amongst nuts, walnuts offer excellent amounts of omega-3 and ratio to omega-6 as well.

Micronutrients

Being plant foods, nuts and seeds are naturally rich in most minerals and vitamins. They are an especially abundant source of minerals like calcium, magnesium, manganese, iron, copper, zinc and selenium. Like other plant foods, their benefits are most powerful for us when we diversify our consumption of them.

Healing & Prevention

In light of their plentiful nutrient content, nuts and seeds play various roles in helping us to maintain healthy bodies that are free of disease and able to heal. The rich source of healthy fats helps to ward off inflammation and heart disease and ensure optimal functioning of all of our cells, tissues, and organs that rely on healthy fats, especially the brain and nervous system. Fats also help in blood-glucose and satiety regulation. This, along with being low in sugars, allows nuts and seeds to help keep our blood sugar levels stable and prevent Type 2 diabetes. The many vitamins, minerals, antioxidants, and phytonutrients in a serving of nuts will enhance all areas of your health, offering cancer and immune system protection. Nuts and seeds also contribute to healthy skin, hair, and nails, as well as longevity.

Nut & Seed Choices for You

The wonderful world of nuts and seeds is also extremely diverse. However, just as we are fixated on wheat, limiting our grains, our society also singled out peanuts and seldom looks elsewhere in the nut category. Peanuts are not truly nuts at all, yet they bear the name and are commonly consumed and considered such. It should come as no surprise that, as with wheat, we are seeing an epidemic of peanut allergies today. My hunch is that, similarly to wheat, modification and chemical treatment of peanuts throughout the decades, an effort to make the crop profitable, may have a lot to do with this. Additionally, the over-consumption of a food is thought to lead to allergies. This makes sense when we consider that wheat and peanuts are amongst the Big-8, a group of the eight major allergenic foods, and all the more reason to diversify our food choices.

Nuts and seeds come in various shapes, sizes, and—best of all—flavors. The most important thing is to consume them in their raw, unroasted form. The heat applied during roasting denatures their healthy fats and proteins and can render them inflammatory and unhealthy for us. Most nuts and seeds also benefit from being soaked and/or sprouted. Examine the list below and find ways to rotate as many varieties as you can as part of your regular diet. I want to emphasize hemp, flax, and chia seeds again; at least one of these seeds should be consumed daily.

Nuts

- Almonds
- Brazil Nuts
- Cashews
- Chestnuts
- Hazelnuts (Filberts)
- Macadamia Nuts
- Peanuts

- Pecans
- Pine Nuts
- Pistachios
- Walnuts

Seeds

- Chia Seeds
- Flax Seeds
- Hemp Seeds
- Poppy Seeds
- Pumpkin Seeds
- Sesame Seeds
- Sunflower Seeds

Practical Tips for Eating Nuts and Seeds

To finish this section, here are some tips for making the most of nuts and seeds in your diet:

1. **Eat nuts and seeds in their raw and natural form (not roasted, salted, or flavored).** Like all plant-based foods, nuts and seeds are healthiest in their natural and wholesome form. Consuming them raw is essential; during the roasting process, nuts can lose up to 15 percent of their naturally occurring oils, and some of their fats can become oxidized and inflammatory in nature. Flavors, salts, or sugars add unnecessary calories, additives, and toxins, all of which have a negative impact on our health.

2. **Soak nuts and some seeds in water for a few hours to make them easier to digest.** Placing nuts or seeds in water for two to twelve hours is normally good to make them easier to digest and more nutritionally robust. Cashews and sunflower seeds benefit from about two hours of soaking, whereas almonds typically require eight to twelve hours. You can soak enough for a desired serving or for several servings; store soaked nuts in the refrigerator. It is best not to soak hemp, chia, or flax seeds. Hemp seeds do not need it and both flax and chia seeds have mucilaginous properties, which make

them gel in the presence of water. In such form, they are commonly used as plant-based egg replacers in recipes or to make all sorts of delicious plant-based puddings and similar foods. Soaked and/or sprouted nuts and seeds can also be dehydrated to offer a dry nut or seed, but with its improved digestibility and nutrition qualities.

3. **Enjoy a variety of different nuts and seeds regularly, as opposed to sticking to only one kind.** Refer to the list in previous section for new additions to your diet.

4. **Go organic as much as possible.**

5. **Enjoy natural nut and seed butters.** Consuming all-natural (with no additives), unsweetened, organic, preferably raw nut and seed butters is also recommended. You can choose to make nut and seed butters at home for optimal freshness and quality with a high-powered blender or food processor. These will allow you to enjoy the benefits of nuts and seeds in a convenient spread or dip form. You can also easily add other whole food ingredients, like raw cacao powder, pure vanilla, or dates, to create chocolate or other flavored wholesome nut or seed spreads.

6. **Get creative with nuts and seeds in your meals.** Nuts and seeds can be easily eaten as snacks on their own or included as part of almost any meal. You can sprinkle some in a salad, curry dish, stir-fry, hot grain cereal, or use them in your green smoothie. You can make homemade nut milks and nut butters, as mentioned above. One of the best things about nuts and seeds is their amazing versatility. Ground, they can serve as the base of rich and creamy homemade sauces, dips, spreads and wholesome, raw desserts.

CHAPTER 12
Minimal Animal Products

We have almost come full circle in our discussion and understanding of what to eat. We have now arrived at a juncture in our journey that provides a pivoting point for your personal transformation. Since birth, the average person has been raised and conditioned to believe that animal products are part of a healthy and complete diet. (In Chapter 20, we will examine how ideas, true or not, spread through societies and become ingrained cultural beliefs over time.) The foods we adopt as children often become part of our identity as we grow up, so it is understandable why some of us get very defensive when there is any talk of reducing or eliminating animal foods or pointing out their shortcomings. Nevertheless, it is undeniable, as we already covered in Chapters 3 and 4, that animal products are not very ideal foods for our health, weight, and modern, sedentary lifestyle, specifically given their present-day quantity, quality, and preparation methods.

A Problem of Quantity

Never in our history have we eaten such a high quantity and a low quality of animal products as we do today. As mentioned in Chapter 3, some people think early humans ate mostly meat, but this implies a limited understanding; our anatomical and physiological nature is much more herbivorous than carnivorous. To date, various cultures around the world have lived and thrived on plant-based and vegetarian diets. Besides a few cultures like the Inuit, who traditionally ate a diet very high in animal fat and protein but also highly raw, our bodies do not seem to be able to tolerate high amounts of animal products for health and longevity. In fact, even though the Inuit appear to have some adaptations for such a diet, research on their health does not conclusively reflect great health or longevity. Dangers of excessive protein, defined when protein makes up more than 35 percent of total energy intake, include toxic levels of

113

amino and ammonia byproducts, hyperinsulinemia, nausea, diarrhea, and, in rare cases, death, such as rabbit starvation syndrome.[1]

As far as we can tell, based on various fields of research, for most of humanity and human history, animal products have been part of a plant-rich diet. Again, we must consider what makes the most sense in regard to our overall anatomy, physiology, practicality, and availability. Historically speaking, we know meat and animal products were most heavily eaten by a small percentage of the wealthiest, most powerful members of society; the majority of commoners only ate meat in small or infrequent quantities. The amount of meat and animal products consumed has also always varied based on geographic location; it is necessary to eat more fat in cold climates and less in warm ones. Of course, with today's modern heating and cooling and nature-disconnected lifestyles, this doesn't really apply to us anymore.

After the Industrial Revolution and the boom of the postwar era of the 1900s, the entire food and economic scene began to change drastically. The world population also grew rapidly, and small family farms were quickly replaced by mega-factory farms. More people were financially better off than ever, suddenly able to eat a plethora of foods, including animal products they had never been able to afford before. With the industrialization of our farms and food supply the availability of animal foods also grew exponentially. Meat and animal products began to be consumed ravenously, as if we were trying to make up for some illusory deprivation of these foods over the years, but there was one problem: We were never meant to eat animal products in the quantities we have come to accept as normal today. If this wasn't clear previously, it is definitely reflected in our poor health and weight today.

The average, modern-day North American tends to heavily consume animal products, independent of climate or even economic status. In fact, highly processed animal foods, like those associated with fast food, are all too often more readily available and less expensive than wholesome, fresh plant foods. Billions of dollars are spent each year to feature prominent advertising and make us aware of that. Most fast food, which so much of the population eats far too regularly and some even consider their main diet, consists of meat, eggs, and dairy. According to data from the Food and Agriculture Organization (FAO), Americans consume 60 percent more meat than Europeans, and since

1971 global meat consumption has tripled! In North America, USDA data shows that between 1970 and 2000, the specific trend per person has included a slight decrease in red meat consumption but an increase in poultry, fish, and, most significantly, cheese consumption.[2] FAO data depicts that as of 2009, Americans are consuming meats in the distribution of 47 percent poultry, 29 percent beef, and 24 percent pork. This means more than half of the meat eaten by Americans is red meat, and data shows that nearly a quarter of it is processed.[3]

Research continues to warn that red meat consumption, especially processed meat products, is strongly tied to increased heart disease, cancer, other chronic diseases, weight problems, and increased mortality. A 2009 Johns Hopkins University study found that those who consumed the most meat consistently ate an average of 700 calories more per day and had a 27 percent greater likelihood of being obese than meat-eaters who consumed the least.[4] As of 2009, even the American Dietetic Association, which was once opposed to vegetarian diets, now maintains that vegetarians exhibit less obesity and lower rates of chronic medical conditions such as heart disease, diabetes, and hypertension. Ultimately, though, beyond any study, organization, or shadow of a doubt, our own lack of health and excess weight should offer enough proof that our unrestrained consumption of animal products is working against us.

Not only is the high quantity of animals bred for consumption destructive to our health, but it is also harmful to the health of our planet. A 2006 UN/FAO report, "Livestock's Long Shadow," has identified the world's rapidly growing beef farming as the greatest threat to the climate, forests, and wildlife. We are destroying forests around the world, clear-cutting them to make room for more animal feedlots. We are polluting lakes and rivers, as slaughterhouses dump millions of pounds of toxic pollutants—primarily nitrogen, phosphorus, and ammonia—into waterways. We are wasting our resources by producing massive amounts of pesticides, synthetic fertilizers, and drugs needed to produce the food for the animals and maintain them; to make matters worse, all of these end up polluting us and our natural resources. We are further polluting the air, land, and water with the waste of the animals, which translates to hundreds of millions of tons of manure annually. To top all this off, the post production of animal foods is often even more environmentally destructive. Today, the choice of whether or not to consume animal products isn't just a matter of health; it is also a serious environmental matter. It can also be considered a matter of social justice and public welfare, given how much food and water is wasted, going to the animals when it could be going directly to humans who are living in poverty worldwide. It is also a matter of ethics, given how inhumanely the animals are treated. This is why, as I shared with you at the start of this book, what we call healthy or consider optimal nourishment must be addressed today in a broader context, taking our modern challenges to heart and mind. Our food choices are highly influential, and as citizens of Planet Earth, we must take personal accountability for that and act and eat responsibility for our own health and the health of our world.

A Problem of Quality

It is essential to recognize that our increased consumption of animal products goes hand in hand with the ever-decreasing quality of these foods. Ethical and environmental issues aside, it is one thing to consume fresh, raw milk from a local cow or meat from a local, organically raised, grass-fed animal, but it is quite another to consume a white, factory-produced beverage called milk or a slab of meat-looking product called chicken, taken from an animal that was unable to hold its own weight within a few weeks of its life due to the unnatural food and drugs it was given. The extent to which you choose to consume animal products on your personal journey of healing and prevention will depend on your personal health and weight needs, your priorities, and your values. However, across the board, our reliance on animal products must decrease and the quality of any animal products we consume must increase if we are truly seeking good health and bodies that can heal and prevent chronic disease. Animal products are acid-forming, devoid of fiber, naturally high in calories and fat, low in many micronutrients, devoid of Vitamin C, and, if not from natural, organic sources, full of various drugs, chemicals, and genetically modified ingredients. Today, we know that not all saturated fat is bad, but the specific fat present in animal foods—a lot of which is saturated—along with some trans fats and cholesterol, appears to have negative effects on our health and weight. Cholesterol alone, something no plant foods contain but animal foods are a source of, is highly problematic for us. In fact, elevated cholesterol appears to be one of the most common lifestyle-related health problems today, leading to further heart disease, chronic diseases, and weight problems.

Cholesterol-lowering statin drugs are among the most commonly prescribed drugs in the U.S.

Animal products are also high in protein; contrary to popular belief, though, this is not necessarily a positive thing. High protein intake, especially from animal products, is associated with liver and kidney problems, bone thinning, and low-grade chronic acidosis; this alone leads to numerous health problems. *Casein*, an animal protein found mostly in dairy, has been linked to cancer promotion. (The mechanisms behind this are outlined in detail in The China Study.[5]) Animal products take a long time to digest and contain no fiber themselves. Eaten as part of a low-fiber diet, they increase chances of constipation, flatulence, digestive problems, and colon cancer. Why the correlation to colon cancer specifically? Because as the animal flesh putrefies in our intestines, various toxins are produced and/or released. If these toxins are not cleared out of our intestines in a timely manner, as is commonly the case with low-fiber diets, they can cause DNA damage, leading to cancer and other health problems. Research has also pointed out that the link between red meat and heart disease goes beyond how lean or how high in fat the meat is; rather, it comes down to the type of bacteria its presence proliferates in our colons. Meat-eaters and non-meat-eaters harbor different intestinal microflora colonies, and these have different impacts on health. A particular bacteria in the human intestines converts a common nutrient found in beef (L-carnitine) into a compound (TMAO) that appears to speed up the buildup of plaque in the arteries.[6]

Apart from the nutrition and health issues, the way modern-day animals are raised and processed is very problematic on its own. Factory-farmed animals are routinely given antibiotics, and these do not magically disappear from the meat when it comes time for us to eat them. The indiscriminate use of antibiotics in our world today, both in humans and animals, has led to various antibiotic resistance problems, increased fungal infections like candida, lack of healthy intestinal flora, various allergies, and other health problems. Given that our world is obsessed with the financial bottom line, we seek to increase production while minimizing costs for every commodity, and this includes animals used for food. Hormones are routinely given to meat, egg, and dairy animals, to make the animals grow unnaturally faster and bigger. Like any drugs, those hormones end up in our bodies. Alarmingly, they have been linked with early onset of puberty in our children and various hormonal imbalances, including elevated estrogen levels in the population, which have ties to breast and other cancers. The addition of hormones to farmed animals is banned in Europe, unlike in North America. As of 1999, the European Union Scientific Committee for Veterinary Measures Relating to Public Health stated that six commonly used growth hormones had the potential to cause endocrine, developmental, immunological, neurobiological, immunotoxic, genotoxic, and carcinogenic effects.

Finally, as animals are higher up on the food chain and high in fat, they have the potential to accumulate toxins in their bodies. Fish and seafood are of the most serious concern, due to the accumulation of mercury and other toxins in our polluted waters today. However, this is not limited to lakes, rivers, and seas; all animals are at risk, given what they are fed and injected with. Modern, factory-farmed animals are given pesticide-sprayed and/or genetically modified feed, as well as foods that are simply not natural for them. Corn, for instance, exposes them and us to a whole host of health problems.

The good news is that organic, naturally raised and fed animals are, for the most part, not subject to the above problems and have much healthier nutritional profiles. One-hundred percent grass-fed beef, for example, has been found to have lower total saturated and monounsaturated fat and more heart-healthy omega-3 fatty acids. This provides us with a lower and healthier ratio of omega-6 to omega-3 fatty acids and higher levels of various micronutrients. The nutritive qualities of organic, raw milk are also starkly different than those of conventional, pasteurized milk. To avoid some of the unpleasant quality problems we have just touched upon, source any meat, eggs, and dairy you choose to consume from local, organic, naturally raised and fed animals, and only consume as part of a high whole plant food/high-fiber diet. If we continue to consume conventional milk, eggs, and meat products found in stores today, whether whole or further processed, we are setting the stage for various health imbalances. Remember that we always have a choice. Even if you don't have easy access to local, organic farms, most stores today offer some organic animal food choices, as do health food stores and farmers' markets. Whether finances are an issue or not, focus on buying a lower quantity and higher quality of animal foods.

A Problem of Preparation

You will recall from Chapter 5 that many problems arise when foods are subjected to high and/or prolonged heat. As we discussed, upon being subjected to high heat and discoloration (browned or blackened from being grilled, barbecued, roasted, or fried) meats produce carcinogenic heterocyclic amines. This is one of several reasons why cultures like the Inuit, who eat high amounts of meat, have an advantage: They eat their meat mostly raw. Pasteurization, a process all commercial dairy is subjected to today, has numerous problems of its own. For starters, pasteurization destroys most of the valuable nutrition benefits of foods, especially enzymes, healthy bacteria, and vitamins. This, in turn, encourages the growth of harmful bacteria in the dairy products and in our intestines. It also biochemically transforms the properties of the original substance, like its sugars, fats, and minerals. For example, pasteurization turns the sugar of milk, lactose, into beta-lactose, which is far more soluble and is, therefore, more rapidly absorbed in the system. It also renders the majority of the milk calcium insoluble, making it unusable for our bodies. Thus, pasteurized dairy has to be fortified with various vitamins and minerals synthetically, and even then, is far from any kind of health food. To add fuel to the fire, the most common cooking and consumption methods of animal foods all too often involve some kind of oil or similar fat, as well as condiments and other processed foods, which are all problematic on their own.

How Much Is Minimal?

"The scientific data is so clear about the fact that eating more than a few small portions of animal products each week is associated with a host of serious diseases."

— Dr. Joel Fuhrman MD, *Eat to Live*

The whole premise of this book is that, in order to enjoy optimal health and wellbeing while optimizing our bodies' natural healing and disease-prevention mechanisms, our diets must be based on whole, natural plant foods. The easiest way to put this into action in a significant way that translates into significantly positive outcomes, without getting bogged down by numbers or calculations, is to revolve your food choices around the three-quarter (75 percent) mark. Aim for a minimum of three-quarters of your food to come from plants, to be alkaline-forming, and to be in its raw form. This means about one-quarter (25 percent) of your daily foods may come from acid-forming and cooked foods, only some of them being animal foods.

Depending on your personal background, you may think this is too restrictive. However, my guidelines are actually much more lenient than what I would recommend from a subjective perspective versus an objective one. There is no doubt in my mind, given the research, as well as my personal and professional experience, that our health, weight, wellbeing, and longevity gain profound benefits the less animal foods there are in our diets—never mind the environmental, ethical, and spiritual benefits. That said, I also understand and respect that everyone is at their own stage of this journey and has their own unique needs and life circumstances, and these must be factored into this equation as well. Therefore, take only the steps you are ready for. At this point, perhaps you could consider eating only one animal product a day, working your way to less than a handful of animal products per week.

Although there are many small- and large-scale scientific studies that illustrate the benefits of a plant-based diet, one of the most notable comes from a large-scale study started in the early 1980s, "The China Study," which lasted over two decades and has a book, with the same title, written about it. According to the experts involved, like Dr. T. Colin Campbell and others who followed in his footsteps, the most significant health benefits (especially heart disease and cancer prevention) were observed when less than 7 to 10 percent of foods came from animal products.[7] As you can imagine, these results made a lot of people very uncomfortable, and various criticisms were put forth, trying to discredit the science. The most critical detail, though, that was overlooked by critics and led to a lot of misunderstanding, was that the study was not based on standard reductionist science principles; rather, it was based on the principles of wholism. I encourage everyone who has any interest in this research to investigate the issue further by reading Dr. Campbell's follow-up book, *Whole: Rethinking the Science of Nutrition*, which comprehensively and elegantly explains the full scope of our modern health, nutrition, and medical landscape and the paradigm shift that is necessary in our society where the science of nutrition is concerned, if we are to succeed in the current nutrition, health, and weight crisis.

As you consider cutting back animal foods to a minimum, apprehensions about insufficient protein and other nutrients may surface for you. This is to be expected, especially given our heavily conditioned ideas about protein. The good news, however, is that by reducing animal products in your diet, you are actually improving your protein intake. Diets high in any nutrient, outside of its most optimal human range, are unhealthy for us; protein included. Given the fact that the body thrives on balance, this should come as no surprise. Furthermore, every whole food, aside from pure sugar and fat, is a source of protein, so protein should be the least of our worries. If you are eating enough food from varied sources each day, even if it is plant foods only, you will easily meet and even exceed your protein requirements. Nature has perfectly designed her foods to sustain and nourish us; you don't have to combine or count anything. Ultimately, as you continue on this journey, it is essential to keep learning and to surround yourself with supportive people and resources that will help you build a solid foundation. This will help you gain certainty about your health and nutrition and make you confident about your choices. In Chapter 17, we will dive deeper into the topic of nutrients and the futile numbers game so many of us are caught up in.

Nutrients & Calories

Animal products are very high in calories, unless they are synthetically defatted. They owe a lot of these calories to their high-fat, high-protein composition. Dairy products tend to be the most deceiving. Many people go for low- or zero-fat dairy products, but these are unnaturally altered, and more often than not, prove to be more harmful to our health and weight than their full-fat counterparts. You may think 2 percent milk is only 2 percent fat, but it actually offers 35 percent of its total calories in fat. Anything over 30 percent is normally considered a high-fat food. If you choose to continue eating multiple animal products regularly, you must be very conscious about how this translates for your health and weight.

To figure out the real content of fat in any packaged food:
1. Multiply the total fat per serving by 9 (1 gram of fat = 9 calories).
2. Divide this number by the total calories of the same serving.
3. Multiply the decimal you get by 100 to get your final fat percentage.

Fiber

Animal foods do not contain any fiber; fiber is only found in plant foods. In fact, animal foods tend to be the most constipating substances and have been linked with colorectal cancer; thus, they should only be eaten as part of an otherwise high-fiber diet.

Macronutrients

Although most people think animal foods are mostly protein, they are actually very high sources of fat. Depending on the food, it can be nearly 50 percent fat and 50 percent protein, so it is somewhat of a fallacy to consider them as "the protein" of a particular meal or diet. Additionally, as we touched upon in earlier chapters, no food is a single nutrient. It may be high in a certain nutrient, but it will also include other nutrients and substances, and those others have the potential to increase or decrease the health value of the food item. We will examine more of these numbers and nutrients in Chapter 17.

Cooked meats generally have no carbohydrates, but dairy has some, normally in the form of sugars. Flavored milk, like chocolate, is actually a very processed food and should be avoided because it is high in sugars and other additives.

Micronutrients

All animal products contain some vitamins and minerals, but they come nowhere close to the nutrient density of plant foods, especially fruits and vegetables. Common animal foods are not a source of Vitamin C, for example, though they do contain some B12. Dairy products are commonly equated with being the go-to source for calcium, to help build healthy bones, but we know today that this story is very incomplete. There are far better sources of bioavailable calcium, like leafy greens, which do not also come with negative health effects. This will be discussed further in Chapter 16. While Vitamin D is present in fish and some dairy products, most of it in dairy comes from fortified, synthetic sources. Finally, animal products are completely devoid of phytonutrients, the powerful healing and preventative compounds that only plants contain; these often come with powerful antioxidant properties, providing us with such benefits as well.

Healing & Prevention

There may still be some conflicting information out there when it comes to animal products, but it is pretty clear that eating animal products is not correlated with reducing the risk of cancer, heart disease, or diabetes, the top three lifestyle diseases, or supporting optimal weight and wellbeing. Aside from meat-oriented diet fads, nearly every piece of medical, health, and nutrition literature echoes the same message: Reduce your consumption of animal products for healing, prevention, good health, and weight.

In terms of healing and prevention benefits, animal products are most notably promoted for their protein, iron (red meat), calcium (dairy), and omega-3 fatty acids (fish). The protein, as mentioned above, is a nonissue. As long as we eat a sufficient amount and variety of food, we are more than easily covered. Animal food producers have played the protein card long enough, but the protein bubble is bursting as people continue to gain a more complete understanding of this nutrient and come to realize that more is far from better. Iron can also be found in many other foods, and it is not guaranteed that those suffering from low iron will benefit by eating red meat or that the high amount of iron in red meat is optimal. There are many biochemical factors involved in the digestion, absorption, storage, and utilization of iron by our bodies. The calcium and dairy connection was mentioned previously in this chapter and other chapters, and we know there are major flaws in the long-spouted dairy-equals-healthy-bones assertion. Thankfully, more of us are realizing that consuming dairy may actually work against rather than for our bone health. Recall that pasteurized dairy is acid-forming, and among the slew of its other problems—allergies, skin conditions, mucus production, and acne, for example—it really is not a compelling food to eat. What we have been conditioned to believe is a far cry from the truth.

Perhaps the greatest nutrition benefits of animal foods that can be easily equated with healing and prevention come from fish. There is no doubt that fish is a source of heart- and brain-healthy, anti-inflammatory omega-3 fats. However, in light of our chemically and radioactively polluted waters, one must seriously weigh the benefits against the disadvantages of consuming today's seafood. Heavy metals, like mercury, as well as other toxins, like polychlorinated biphenyls (PCBs), readily accumulate in the fatty tissues of fish. Fish from various areas of the Pacific Ocean also carry a radioactive risk. Farmed fish have their own problems, similar to those of factory-farmed animals, and we can no longer depend on our formerly pristine lakes and rivers; today, they are home to all sorts of chemical concoctions. Therefore, even eating fish today has become a highly controversial, personal matter that must be examined in light of all the tradeoffs. If you are a middle-aged man, there may be more benefits than risks for you; on the other hand, if you are a young female who intends to get pregnant, there are probably more risks than benefits.

Ultimately, we must factor in the overall quality of one's diet and lifestyle to better assess any risks or benefits of eating seafood. Carefully research the fish you are interested in eating, as they each have higher or lower concentrations of toxic pollutants based on their type and the geographical location they are sourced from. The Natural Resources Defense Council (NRDC) has created an online calculator (see link below) consumers can freely use to check the level of mercury consumed and what risks this translates to based on your weight and the type of seafood, portion size, and number of portions consumed. We will cover more about fish, fish oils, omega-3, and algae (where the fish get their omega-3 fatty acids) in Chapter 16, when we discuss supplements. For the meantime, know that diets based on natural, whole, plant foods, especially greens, are often more protective and balanced in omega-3 and omega-6 fatty acids than most people realize. We do not need to get caught up in consuming fish, specialty oils, or supplements to benefit our body in optimal ways. We can benefit more by reducing and removing the destructive culprits from our diet, like processed foods, along with their various inflammation-inducing oils, and high amounts of animal products.

> **NRDC Mercury Calculator for Seafood**
> www.nrdc.org/health/effects/mercury/calculator/calc.asp

Today, it is quite tricky to eat animal products safely and in any healthy fashion. Whether you choose to include some in your diet or not is not really the issue; in the end, this is up to you. The main point is that for optimal health, proper healing, and prevention against all disease, we must base our diets on whole, natural plant foods. We must also understand that animal products are not a mandatory part of that. When approached properly, a 100 percent plant-food diet may offer the best benefits for weight loss, healthy weight maintenance, and prevention and healing of the diseases we face today.

Practical Tips for Eating Animal Products

To finish this section, here are some tips for making the most of eating animal products in the healthiest way possible:

1. **If you choose to eat any dairy, the healthiest choice is organic, all-natural, fermented dairy, such as plain kefir or yogurt.** Avoid commercial, processed, and flavored yogurt. We will cover this further in Chapter 14.

2. **If you choose to drink milk, research raw milk from local, organic farmers.** If you must use store-bought milk, only consider organic. You may also wish to consider goat over cow milk; it has a nutrient profile that is slightly better suited for us and several other advantages over cow milk.

3. **Avoid all cheese.** It is the most problematic dairy food when it comes to our health and weight. Cheese contains the highest concentration of casein, fat, and cholesterol and is addictive and highly acid-forming. Casein, the milk protein we touched upon earlier that is linked with promoting cancer, is found in extremely high levels in cow's milk. It is most concentrated in cheese and is responsible for the addictive qualities, as during digestion it is capable of breaking down into *casomorphin*, an opioid compound.

4. **If you choose to eat fish, focus on deep, cold-water ocean fish.** Research the type of fish you are interested in eating, where it comes from, and the

relative risk associated with its consumption. Use the NRDC calculator I shared with you earlier in this chapter to calculate your levels of mercury. Choose unprocessed fresh or frozen fish only.

5. **If you choose to eat any meat, focus on local, pasture raised, grass-fed, lean, organic meat.** As to whether beef, chicken, or pork is the healthiest option, they all have their own pros and cons. Scientifically speaking, red meat does have the strongest link to chronic disease and weight problems. Avoid factory-farmed, grain-fed, and processed meats at all costs.

6. **If you choose to eat eggs, focus on eggs from local, organic, and naturally fed and raised birds.**

7. **Avoid grilling, roasting, barbecuing, or frying meat, fish, and eggs.** Opt for boiled or steamed options, and avoid eating any blackened or burned animal food parts.

CHAPTER 13
Water & Other Drinks

We have almost completed our journey into understanding optimal food choices for healing and prevention of disease and optimal health. Before we finish, we need to discuss beverages and drinks, beyond the green smoothies and dairy options we've already mentioned. In this section, we will talk about these, water in particular, as it should be our prime fluid of choice. Water may not be considered a food, since it is not eaten and carries no calories, but it is essential for optimal health, weight, healing, and prevention.

While there has been a resurgence in water's popularity in the last few decades, especially with the emergence of bottled water, many people are still not drinking enough of this highly valuable substance. Most people rely on coffee, tea, juice beverages, energy drinks, and sodas for their main intake of daily fluids. This is unfortunate, because none of these can adequately replace water. In fact, many of these beverages have a diuretic effect, encouraging the body to excrete water through urination rather than retain it. Additionally, these are a source of unnecessary, empty calories, various additives, synthetic nutrients, sugars, caffeine, and other unfavorable ingredients.

When we are told that we need to drink water each day, in a certain amount, we may falsely assume that all liquids count. This is simply not the case. While other liquids may help with hydration, they can also mask true thirst and deceive us into thinking we are hydrated. Besides, the reason for taking in water goes well beyond hydration. In fact, we need to drink more water just to counteract the effects of beverages like coffee and caffeinated tea.

Our bodies are comprised of over 70 percent water, and water is required for almost all of the thousands of reactions, processes, and functions that have to take place in our bodies daily. Most of us are not aware that the majority of the population is chronically dehydrated. This is not just surface-level dehydration, in which one feels thirsty all the time; rather, it is a deep-level dehydration, forcing the body to cope with a smaller than optimal amount of water on a regular basis. Some people find this hard to believe and argue that if we were thirsty or dehydrated, our bodies would let us know. The fact is that so many of us are so out of tune with our bodies and have bodies that are so out of balance that we cannot easily depend on even the most basic signals. We eat when we are not hungry, drink when we are not thirsty, and often mistake thirst for hunger. Additionally, when we fill our ourselves with other foods or drinks, we have no desire for water, even though our bodies might be greatly in need of it. There is only so much room, after all, and when we fill our stomachs with the wrong stuff, we leave no room for what we truly need.

Common symptoms of chronic dehydration include fatigue, constipation, headaches, joint pain, digestive imbalances, blood pressure imbalances, acid-alkaline imbalance, and premature aging. Chronic dehydration can also cause histamines to become excessively active. This may result in symptoms that mimic various allergies and can be mistaken for other disorders, such as asthma or even colitis. Chronic dehydration is also not something that can be fixed overnight by drinking more water; it takes time and requires a regular and sufficient intake of pure water.

Water is necessary to flush toxins out of the body, and it is one of the best detox substances we have. It is the number-one lubricant within and ensures proper functioning of all cells, tissues, and organs. All of our bodily fluids and internal cell environments are based on water. It hydrates cells, is necessary for proper skin elasticity, and decreases wrinkles. It is the number-one solvent within our bodies, for beneficial and harmful substances alike. Ultimately, I don't have to convince you that water is critical not only to our health but to our very lives; we all know we would die within a few days without it.

While many of us have taken the water message seriously in recent years, a great many are still not getting enough pure water regularly enough. We fill up on processed beverages, and there are some who literally never drink pure, unflavored, unprocessed water. Aside from our innate calling that naturally drives us to seek pure water, learning about its importance can be a great motivator to take its consumption seriously. When I learned what we know academically today about the multifactorial power of water, I honestly could not see having room to drink anything but water! Just to be fair, though, let's take a quick look at other beverages to see if they have any value for the creation and maintenance of an optimally healthy body.

Other Liquid Drinks

Commercial juices are really a form of sugar water, even when they are unsweetened. Whatever natural benefits might have come from the fruits are pretty much lost during their processing and pasteurization. They easily contribute to blood-glucose imbalances, as they are missing the valuable fiber found in whole fruit and are a source of extra calories. The packaging they sit in for days, weeks, or months is usually plastic, so it has its own problems. Don't be fooled into thinking they are good sources of Vitamin C or calcium; these are synthetically added and can be easily and most naturally found in whole fruits and vegetables. The only fruit drink that is suitable for optimal health is pure, fresh juice from various vegetables and fruits, preferably home-juiced or blended with water for a smoothie. More about this will be discussed in Chapter 19.

Artificial beverages, energy drinks, and soda are completely synthetic, processed foods. That, coupled with their sugar-loaded, chemical properties, means they have no place in the diet of anyone who is serious about their weight and health. They are a source of refined sugars, artificial colors, flavors, additives, and chemicals. Sugar-free varieties, sweetened with toxic, artificial sweeteners, have been linked to numerous serious health problems, including preterm delivery for pregnant women.[1] They are a waste of your money, health, and environmental resources. Part of becoming optimally healthy is also becoming optimally aware of how each of our choices contributes to the food and healthcare system we have allowed to dominate versus the one we wish to create.

Vitamin water is an insult to both water and vitamins. It is amazing what clever marketing can do and how we fall for it if we are not mindful. Drinking synthetic, isolated vitamins, especially on an empty stomach, greatly diminishes and defeats their purpose. Synthetic, isolated nutrients will never be able to compete with wholesome, natural nutrients, nor will they create optimal wellbeing. Again, we will discuss this more in Chapter 16. The quality and effects of so-called filtered water used in such drinks, which then sits in plastic bottles, will be covered in the next section. To date, vitamin water has been exposed for what it is, a synthetic substance and sugar water at best.

Type 2 diabetes is reaching epidemic proportions today, and it is one of the three main lifestyle diseases that is afflicting North Americans. Diabetes does not mean one will simply die prematurely or be healed after some major surgery. This debilitating disease unfolds over decades, starting with a mild loss in the quality of life and becoming progressively worse over time. It confines most to pharmaceutical dependence and unnatural food restrictions. The good news is that this does not have to be our reality. In comparison to heart disease and cancer, Type 2 diabetes is the most easily preventable disease, and you can almost guarantee that you will not suffer from it if you make the right lifestyle choices. It is so empowering to know that it is completely within our control to prevent ourselves from ever having diabetes and several other health conditions, and avoid suffering and pain in our future just by making different food and drink choices today.

Sugary drinks, like soda, cause rapid spikes in our blood-glucose. This puts a strain on our pancreas and insulin balance. Chronically elevated insulin levels, a common side effect of a diet high in refined carbohydrates and sugary drinks, lead to insulin resistance and are a foundational factor of most chronic disease, from diabetes to cancer. Isolated, refined sugars are inflammatory, acid-forming, and easily converted into fat, leading to excess weight. One of the biggest culprits in most sugary drinks is an unnaturally high, refined fructose content. After World War II, the food industry began to incorporate high fructose corn syrup (HFCS) into many common foods and drinks, mainly because it was cheaper and sweeter than sucrose sugar. For decades, many people had no idea that the type of sugar we consume made any difference; today, however, most of us understand and agree that there is a big difference. Refined, synthetic, and isolated fructose has a far different effect on us than natural, whole, food-bound fructose, such as that that naturally occurs in fruit. Refined fructose, like HFCS, is more chemically reactive than glucose. It circulates in the blood at a much lower concentration, and because it cannot enter most cells, it is primarily metabolized by the liver. Some experts have even gone so far as to call it a toxin or a poison, based on the incredible liver damage it is capable of causing. This only leads to other imbalances and diseases. A publication in the *American Journal of Clinical Nutrition* also presents the correlation associated with the intake of soft drinks containing high-fructose corn syrup or sucrose to the epidemic of obesity in both adults and children.[2] We will examine fructose in further in Chapter 14.

Coffee

Coffee is one of the most heavily consumed beverages in North America and one that can also be highly destructive to our health. The majority of the population suffers from such extreme energy imbalances that they cannot function properly without this stimulant, and many are heavily addicted. Thus, it can be uncomfortable or even provocative to talk about how unsavory coffee really is when it comes to optimal health. For many people, this addiction, or habit as many like to call it, is as taxing to the wallet as it is to their health. It does not help either that studies on coffee are often quite conflicting, citing some benefits that seem to only encourage people to further justify this habit. As with all headlines and studies though, we have to look below the surface to properly assess any real or potential value. There is no doubt that coffee does have some potential benefits. As a natural, whole plant food, it is a source of some nutrients and antioxidants, but it is also a source of some powerful medicinal compounds. The problems associated with coffee revolve around these compounds, as well as how it is industrially grown with various synthetic fertilizers and pesticides, what we do with the bean during processing, what we add to the beverage itself, and the unnatural quantities we consume. When we consider the pros and cons of coffee in light of its most common usage, it offers much more harm than good. It is an addictive substance that alters brain function, including mood. It has a negative effect on our adrenal glands, distorts our energy levels, and increases the risk of adrenal fatigue syndrome. It is highly acid-forming and is, thus, disastrous for bone health, increasing the risk of osteoporosis and inflammation among other things. Coffee interferes with the body's ability to use folate and Vitamins B12 and B6. It stains the teeth, can exacerbate acid indigestion, and causes sleep problems, as caffeine can loiter in the system for up to twelve hours. It can raise our cholesterol, cause insulin irregularities, and increase the risk of heart disease and blood pressure, even causing occasional irregular heartbeat. Keep in mind that what I am sharing here is also a very short and simplified summary of coffee's possible side-effects. Ultimately, there really is no benefit from consuming coffee that one cannot get elsewhere, particularly none that is worth all the risks.

When the coffee bean was used by indigenous people, its quality and quantity was very different from what we drink today. Nature provides powerful substances that can aid in healing and prevention, but we need to respect and know how to use them rather than abuse them. We are quite disconnected from nature in our modern society, so we often undermine the medicinal properties of plants, not realizing that they can have powerful effects that can heal or harm. Such is the case with coffee. It is an amazingly potent collection of biologically active compounds, with caffeine being just one tiny part and making up a mere one to two percent of the bean. The intricate roles of the many other compounds need further study, but for proper use and health outcomes, coffee should be treated more like a drug than any type of food or beverage.

If you are like many people in the population, the idea of giving up coffee leaves you cringing, perhaps even getting defensive. I've commonly been asked what minimum amount is safe to consume. The answer is that there is no one, magic number. It will have a different effect and risk potential for each individual and depend on your overall state of health, diet, and other lifestyle habits. If you are eating highly alkaline regularly with minimal to no processed food, exercising, sleeping well, and not ingesting other harmful substances, then perhaps a cup or two per week won't be a big deal. However, things get complicated if you are already suffering from a condition, if you experience high stress levels on a regular basis, or if you have unhealthy lifestyle habits. You may be tempted to turn to decaf, but that can actually be even more harmful, since it is chemically processed. To remove caffeine from coffee, a chemical solvent such as trichloroethylene or the more popular methylene chloride is used, and neither of these is at all good for your health. If you do choose to consume any coffee, do your best to ensure that it comes from the purest, high-quality, organic sources. Consume it black (plain, without any dairy or sweeteners), and drink it in small quantities, infrequently.

Tea

When it comes to tea, the discussion can go both ways. Herbal teas tend to be alkaline-forming, whereas regular tea tends to be acid-forming. Herbal teas that are naturally free of caffeine and do not include any additives can be very beneficial in many ways for healing, prevention, weight loss, and wellbeing. They can be used medicinally and are a great addition to an optimally healthy lifestyle. If you enjoy tea or warm beverages, feel free to explore and experience the abundant variety of herbal teas. Of course it is best to enjoy them plain, without the addition of any sweeteners or dairy products. Also, if you buy herbal tea blends, always check the ingredients for any added flavors or other unnecessary ingredients.

Green tea is a good source of antioxidants and has been linked to many positive health benefits. However, keep in mind that green tea does contain some caffeine. The good news is that green tea has about a third of the caffeine as coffee, and it also has other beneficial compounds that are known to help neurotransmitter balance, promote natural detoxing and healthy digestion, and can counteract some of the effects of caffeine. It can definitely be a valuable addition to an optimally healthy diet, but it is in no way a necessary one.

Regular tea borders on the side of coffee; again, while some benefits exist, the drawbacks are of a greater importance. Common dairy and sweetener additions don't help. For optimal healing and prevention, it is best to avoid regular tea and stick with green tea or herbal tea instead.

Alcohol

When it comes to alcohol, it reminds me very much of coffee; there are many claims about this or that benefit, yet it has so many known negative health consequences. First, there are different types of alcohol, from the absolute worst (chemically flavored, sweetened, and colored alcoholic beverages) to the best of the worst (organic red wine). While red wine may be touted in a study or claim to be beneficial to our health in some way, allow me to clarify something: Alcohol is a neurotoxin. This means that it negatively affects your neurons, your brain cells, every time, with no exceptions, and it adds more stress to your liver in a day and age where that overtaxed organ likely has enough to deal with. In fact, the National Toxicology Program of the U.S. Department of Health and Human Services lists the consumption of alcoholic beverages as a known human carcinogen. We must also understand that alcohol is rich in calories and loaded with unfavorable carbohydrates. Next to fat, it is the second richest source of calories, coming in at seven calories per gram, yet nutritionally worthless. Thus, it is neither health-friendly nor weight-friendly.

Alcohol is also especially destructive to women's health. Women break the substance down more slowly than men, giving the toxin more time to inflict damage. Alcohol use in women has been connected with various negative effects, including increased risk of heart disease, sleep problems, depression, and breast cancer.[3] I could list all the other negative ways alcohol affects every part of your body, male or female, but if you are serious about your health and are reading this book, I am hoping I don't have to convince you any further. If you would like the details, though, there are plenty of books and articles that explore these destructive qualities in detail.

Alcohol is also one of those things that goes far beyond being merely a health concern. It is also a major societal concern. Commercials tout that we should "enjoy responsibly," but the truth of the matter is that we cannot even enjoy our food responsibly, never mind a substance that alters our physical, mental, and emotional state so radically. As I mentioned to you at the beginning of this book, this journey is not about making excuses or passively following the status quo. It is about taking a stand for what you believe in, and, as such, I cannot support or promote, in any amount, a substance so highly addictive and destructive, one that alters our mind, distorts our awareness, and impairs our ability to be a highly functioning human being.

I understand that, for some of us, it is a matter of flavor. For others, it is a form of stress release, and for some it is just a social thing or simply just a habit. Whatever your reasons, the choice remains yours, and you must follow your personal priorities. One of the things I am aiming to do is to help you strengthen your muscle of personal accountability. We've become so used to hearing how much of this or that we should be eating or drinking and have resorted to living based on external guidance, when the best guidance should come from within. It is not about one or two drinks per day, per week, or that erroneous "in moderation." There are no magic, one-size-fits-all numbers for healthy alcohol consumption, and general guidelines only go so far. When something goes wrong, *we* have to deal with the consequences, and it does us little good to lay external blame. There are certain substances, with alcohol being one of them, which have the odds stacked against them when it comes to creating health, and when we choose to consume them we are gambling with very high stakes. I therefore invite you to look beyond the media, the social correctness, and your upbringing and connect with your inner guidance system to decide what is truly best for you. If you use alcohol as any kind of escape tool, my advice is to open yourself up to engaging more fully and authentically with life. Pursue a journey of self-discovery, self-love and self-fulfillment. Learn to get high on life rather than on harmful, biochemically altering substances.

But what about all the known health benefits of red wine? To be fair, we must answer that question before we fully leave this topic. For starters, research is inconclusive as to whether red wine really has more benefits than any other alcohol when it comes to possibly being protective against heart disease. All alcohol, by its very nature, can dilute or thin blood, reducing the build up of plaque and risk of blood clots. These benefits however, offer a type of band-aid solution and even then for a very small percentage of the population who would be deemed to get more benefit, than harm from regular, minimal alcohol consumption. The real solution is to change the diet and lifestyle to be naturally protective, rather than destructive. When it comes to red wine specifically, it has a high concentration of polyphenol phytonutrients with antioxidant properties called flavonoids. Some of red wine's main benefits come from another polyphenol found in red grapes, resveratrol, which also has antioxidant properties, as well as anti-cancer and anti-inflammatory properties. But here is the funny part: According to the Mayo Clinic, animal studies to date show that you would need to drink over 60 liters a day, about 100 bottles of red wine, to get the dose of resveratrol needed to show the supposed health benefits.[4] Red grapes, especially when organic and eaten with seeds, have the highest natural concentration of resveratrol. From that perspective, if you want the health benefits of resveratrol, it seems much more efficient and logical to go directly to the source, the red grape. Bottom line, alcohol can in no way replace a healthy diet or offer something that a healthy diet and lifestyle cannot. It will however introduce lots of stress and possible damage to the body, every single time.

All Water Is Not Created Equal

At the end of the day, if you want optimal health and weight, and a body that knows how to properly heal and protect itself from disease, there is no going about it without water. As I mentioned above, we could continue to drink the other beverages if they at least added to our health more benefit than harm, but they don't. Apart from home-juicing and herbal teas, the other beverages contribute more problems than advantages where our health is concerned.

When it comes to picking the best water for optimal health, we must also realize that all water is not created equal. Just as there is processed food, there is processed water. The most beneficial water for optimal health is pure, natural spring water that comes from the deep, free-flowing springs in nature. Visit www.findaspring.com for a directory of local springs all over the world, and see what you may have available in your area. The next best thing may be water from a deep well, if you have access to a high-quality source of such water. For most of us, however, the best water will come from properly filtered tap water. There are many filters to choose from today, some very inexpensive and others a significant investment. Research and learn what may be right for your home and water quality needs.

One of the popular sources of water to minimize your use of and entirely avoid if possible is bottled water. While this fad has hooked many people over the past two decades, it is a huge waste of financial and environmental resources, not to mention that it fails to provide a convincingly better quality of water. The majority of bottled water comes from questionable municipal sources, with some form of basic filtration. Not only is it bottled in plastic, where it can sit in warm environments, including direct sunlight for significant periods of time, but various problems have been discovered with respect to its bacterial, pollutant, and toxin levels. Bottled water is not tested like municipal water, and any testing that is done is not necessarily reflective of the product by the time it reaches you. Unless you find yourself in a foreign country, where you may have to depend on bottled water, save your money, the environment, and your health and choose otherwise. Water is a basic right that should be free for all; it should not be a profit-making venture.

The only bottled water that may be worth buying occasionally is real mineral water (not Perrier or other carbonated water). This means water that has come from real, artesian springs, without any filtration or processing. As the name implies, it is naturally rich in minerals like calcium and magnesium and has an alkalizing effect. High-quality water like this will typically come in a glass bottle. Such water is normally sourced from mineral-rich springs found throughout Europe, in Italy, Germany, or Poland. Of course, the health benefits have to be weighed against the financial and environmental drawbacks. It can be a great choice if you are somewhere where you need to depend on bottled water, but not necessarily as your daily choice.

When it comes to tap water, the quality varies greatly, depending on where you live. While some regions or municipalities offer decent tap water, most supply chlorinated, fluoridated water with various pharmaceuticals, toxins, and other impurities. If you drink mostly from the tap, you need a decent filter. The dangers of fluoride are more commonly known today, and it is never a good idea to consume toxins. Many communities are working on removing fluoride from their municipal water supply, and numerous organizations continue to bring awareness to its dangers, like the Flouride Action Network at fluoridealert.org

Nutrients & Calories

Water does not contain any calories or vitamins. It has some minerals, depending on the source, and some mineral water is an excellent source of calcium and magnesium. Since water has no calories, it has no carbohydrates, fats, or proteins.

Healing & Prevention

As mentioned in the introduction of this chapter, water is critical for every aspect of good health. Every single cell, tissue, and organ depends on water for proper functioning. Water helps to optimize the brain, the liver, the immune system, and the digestive system; ensure proper elimination, detox, and cleansing; aid in weight loss and healthy weight maintenance; and promote optimal wellbeing.

How Much Water Is the Right Amount?

Over the years, there have been various answers to this question. From this many cups to that many liters, these variations in advice have left some of us quite confused. The fact is that many variables influence how much water one needs. Even for an individual person, the amount can vary daily based on the state of activity, environmental temperature, food eaten that day, state of health, stress level, etc. Therefore, it is best to self-regulate by listening to your body, though this is not always the most reliable way for everyone to go.

While we have heard in the past that we should drink 6 to 8 glasses of water, this makes most sense if we are assuming a glass to be about 250 ml or 8 ounces. That quantity would then equate to 1.5 to 2 liters (48 to 64 ounces) of water daily, which is a smart guideline to follow.

Another way to estimate the amount of water needed, and a little more specific to meet individual needs, is by using the following equation:

Take your weight in pounds and divide it by two. Switch the units to ounces (no conversion needed). This is the optimally recommended amount of water for your weight.

For example, if someone weighs 200 pounds, when we divide it by 2, we get 100 pounds. Switching the units to ounces means we would need 100 ounces, or 3 liters (1 oz = 30 ml), of water per day.

Ultimately, drinking water should not be a chore or a complicated math equation. Simply have high-quality water readily available around you and regularly sip it throughout the day. Any obsessive-compulsive behavior can work against us, so don't make a sport of drinking water. Also, try to avoid drinking it while eating or directly after eating. Digestion works best when we do not dilute our digestive juices and enzymes. This may take some time to adjust, depending on your habits up until now, but it is of the utmost value for optimal digestion and wellbeing. Focus on food when it is time to eat, and enjoy water's numerous benefits throughout the other parts of your day.

CHAPTER 14
Other Foods

Along our journey into optimal nutrition for healing and prevention, we have rediscovered the power of real, whole foods like fruits, vegetables, nuts, seeds, grains, and beans. Before we wrap up our focus on food, there are a few others I would like to touch upon to help you understand their role in creating your health and how to optimize their use.

Oils

As a society we have become very reliant on oils for our cooking and food preparation needs, even in the healthiest of diets. The very first thing, though, to understand about oils is that they are all processed in one way or another, and they provide us with a very isolated nutrient and unnatural food. Nature provides whole foods, rich in a variety of macro- and micronutrients, not isolated nutrients. Pure fat—just like pure sugar—is something we have created by processing our foods. Most of us can easily deduce today that isolated or refined sugar is an extremely unhealthy substance; rich in calories, devoid of nutrients, and harmful for our health in a myriad of ways. We have yet to apply this same logic to the oils. We have made some isolated nutrients work for us, but more often than not, consuming nutrients in isolated forms ends up working against us. Of course, the methods by which the foods are processed will have a big impact on their quality and subsequent health effects. When it comes to oils, we have to be very diligent about understanding them and using them in the most appropriate ways.

Whether for cooking or in raw form, most of us want some kind of oil in our diet. Most whole-food, plant-based experts, however, advise against all oils for healing, prevention, and optimal health. Where does that leave you? It will, as always, all depend on your personal health and weight needs, priorities, and choices. If you choose to include any oils in your diet, a few factors must be considered in order to optimize their use. For starters, whole foods that are rich in fats are in no way equivalent to oils that are pure fat. Whole foods include a wide array of macro- and micronutrients. Oils only provide the fat macronutrient and trace amounts, if any, of micronutrients. They are incredibly dense in energy; one gram of fat provides nine calories, the highest quantity of all nutrients. For further reference, roughly one tablespoon of oil provides 120 calories. An optimally healthy, active individual may be just fine if they include some oils in their diet, where as a sedentary, overweight, or disease inflicted individual would not. We must also factor in the quality of the entire diet, as well as the quality of the particular oil. Ideally, you want to drastically limit or entirely avoid all oil, unless there is some specific condition for which a particular oil may prove advantageous. We have to understand that while fat is essential for proper health, healing, and prevention, oils are not. In order to help you be a wise and discerning consumer when it comes to oils, in the next section I will share with you the basics of optimal oil use.

Oil processing falls into one of two categories: *refined* or *unrefined*. Refined oils are mechanically and/or chemically processed to extract the oil and make it suitable for the market. Similar to the grain processing we talked about in Chapter 10, this is mainly done to ensure a longer, more stable shelf life. We know today that refined oils are in no way optimal for our health, and in fact, are extremely destructive to our health. They are typically very mild, if not entirely devoid of taste and aroma. Any trace nutrients they may have had are denatured, if not downright destroyed, and they tend to be highly acid-forming, cell damaging, and inflammatory. Unrefined oils, on the other hand, are processed mechanically or even by hand, typically using lower heat during the extraction process, if any at all. Unrefined oils are normally labelled as virgin or extra-virgin. While saturated fats are the most stable, polyunsaturated ones are the least stable and are easily damaged by heat, light, and oxygen. To maintain their nutritional integrity and any beneficial properties, special care must be taken during the extraction and production process of all oils, especially those rich in polyunsaturated fats. Unrefined oils retain some natural flavor and aroma of the original food from which they come, and they may be a source of some fat-soluble vitamins, antioxidants, and phytonutrients.

All refined oils should be avoided at all costs. As always, read all ingredient lists of any packaged foods that you choose to buy and be mindful of the food choices you encounter when eating out. The healthiest way to consume any unrefined oils is in their natural, raw form. This means on salads, in smoothies, in raw desserts, or added to food after cooking. This way, we will preserve the natural properties and avoid any degradation of the oil. Most unrefined oils, like hemp, flax, evening primrose, and pumpkin seed oil must never be subjected to any heat. When it comes to olive oil, to optimize its use you should also only use it in its raw form and not for cooking.

Many people commonly wonder or ask about the best oil for cooking purposes. Before we answer this question, we must address the cooking aspect itself. As you may recall from Chapter 5, there is great importance to eating food in its most natural, raw form for most healing and prevention benefits. We should not need to know the healthiest oil to fry our food in therefore, as the whole process of frying defeats the purpose of healthy to begin with. If dealing with such culinary practices, I would say it really does not matter which oil you choose, as no oil in the world is going to make such a meal healthy in any way, and definitely not when subjected to extreme heat as well. While some light sautéing, steaming, or stir-frying can be a healthy option, exposing food to high or prolonged heat is never a good idea. Second, after years of research into this subject within the changing field of nutritional science, I have also come to understand that no liquid oil is truly safe to heat. Liquid oils composed of various ratios of monounsaturated and polyunsaturated fats should simply not be exposed to heat. In the past, many people referenced the smoke point of oils as a guide for safe cooking. Today, we know that this cannot be depended on for optimal health reasons, as many oils begin to break down and oxidize before they ever reach their smoke point. The main health risks associated with heated, oxidized, denatured, or refined oils include them being highly inflammatory and causing DNA damage due to the free radicals that are generated. This, amidst our heavy oil use today, is a clear contributor to our unprecedented levels of obesity, heart disease and cancer.

As mentioned, the most stable fats, which tend to be able to handle heat, are saturated fats. Within this category, we are limited to two groups: tropical oils and animal fat. When it comes to animal fat, like lard or butter, I definitely cannot recommend either for numerous reasons, as previously addressed. This leaves us with tropical oils. For many years, all saturated fats were vilified as a major contributing factor to heart disease. Today, we know that our oversimplified and misdirected approach did not serve us well. There are many types of saturated fatty acids, and the different compositions play an integral role in the state of our health. For example, saturated fats from plant sources have different fatty acid profiles than those from animal sources, not to mention come in a completely different whole food package. When it comes to tropical oils, one in particular stands out as an option that may be worthy of our consideration: coconut oil. Research about this oil continues to emerge, though, it is not fully conclusive; it really depends on whose interpretation you get. Native cultures, who have traditionally used coconut oil in its most natural form, have seemed to thrive, without the expected cardiovascular problems associated with saturated fat. There is a critical aspect as to why this may be though that is relevant to olive oil's popularity as well. When looked at from a broader perspective, coconut oil is not the health secret of the Polynesian or South Asian cultures, just like olive oil is not of the Mediterranean cultures. What they both share in common are diets that are based on wholesome, natural, plant foods, rich in fruits and vegetables, which we know today are for certain the most protective and healing for our health. Still, proponents of coconut oil share that it possesses healing properties far beyond that of any other dietary oil. This may very well be true, but it should not be interpreted to mean that you can consume any quality or quantity of it indiscriminately. Only choose unrefined or virgin, organic coconut oil and use sparingly, unless otherwise directed for your personal health needs. When it comes to other tropical oils, they vary in their fatty acid profiles and most are tainted with serious sustainability issues, so they are not recommended.

Although it may already be obvious, I would also like to specifically emphasize some oils that should be avoided at all costs if you are interested in optimal health, weight, healing, and prevention. These include canola, corn, soy, sunflower, safflower, cottonseed, and vegetable oil. The varying problems associated with them include that most of them come from genetically modified organisms, are typically refined, are inflammatory, are high in polyunsaturated fats and prone to oxidation, are too high or excessive in omega-6 fatty acids and too low or devoid of omega-3 fatty acids, and are not stable in heat. This translates to all sorts of stress for our bodies and a cache of grim health problems, including high levels of inflammation and oxidative stress. While you may not purchase them directly, be especially mindful of any processed food or eat-out food, as nearly all processed and common, restaurant foods include them.

PRACTICAL TIPS FOR OIL USE:

1. Oils are not a necessary part of a health-promoting diet. Focus on whole-food, healthy fat sources instead, like raw nuts and seeds, coconuts, olives, and avocados.

2. Any oils you choose to consume should be purchased in their most natural, unrefined (virgin or extra virgin, depending on the oil), and highest-quality versions.

3. Don't cook with liquid (unsaturated) oils. Either use a small amount of virgin coconut oil or simply water to steam, sauté, or stir-fry.

4. Use any oils very sparingly, if at all.

Herbs & Spices

Herbs and spices are extremely healthy and can be liberally added to any dish you choose. They are rich in various vitamins, minerals, phytonutrients, and antioxidants, and they can add plenty of robust flavors to any meal. A bowl of steel-cut oats, or a similar breakfast grain, benefits from some cinnamon, for example, an amazing source of antioxidants. Lunch and dinner meals can both include unique combinations of the wide array of herbs and spices, including optimally healthy turmeric, coriander, oregano, black pepper, cayenne, saffron, tarragon, rosemary, thyme, cumin, sage, basil, and more!

To maximize their numerous health benefits, they should be used in their fresh or dried state. Avoid herbs or spices packaged as specialized dish mixtures, since other additives or preservatives are used. Remember to always read the ingredients, as sugars or MSG and other preservatives may be lurking in there. Choose minimally processed, pure herbs and spices of the highest quality, organic whenever possible.

If you don't have much experience working with herbs and spices, begin with a few and slowly experiment with their flavors. The key is to start by adding a little, a dash or parts of a teaspoonful, and going from there, based on your taste bud preferences. The best way to learn is by allowing yourself to get creative in the kitchen. Some herbs and spices are very forgiving, like basil, oregano, or cinnamon, while others, like turmeric and nutmeg, are not. At first, remember that less is more; it is always easy to add more, but it is far tougher to mask a strong, pungent flavor.

Condiments & Salad Dressings

All bottled condiments, sauces, and dressings are considered processed food and are not included in an optimally healthy diet. They contain numerous additives, preservatives, genetically modified ingredients, sugars, oils, and way too much sodium.

On the other hand, *homemade* salsa, relish, hummus, salad dressings, dips, or other sauces can be a wonderful whole-food, nutrient-dense addition to many meals. They are normally very fast and easy to make with the right blender or food processor (more on this in Chapter 18). Some fresh lemon juice alone does wonders for most salads and any vegetable-based dishes. Add to that some ginger or garlic, and a few herbs or spices and enjoy an abundance of rich and savory flavors. To make any of your sauces or dressings creamy, simply add in a nut or seed; cashews make an exceptionally great choice.

Sweeteners

While we want to reduce, if not entirely eliminate, our usage of all isolated sweeteners, I am happy to share that there is a way to be optimally healthy and enjoy some added sweetness too. As mentioned previously, all sugar is not created equal when it comes to its effect on our health. There are various single, double-, and multiple sugars that belong to the carbohydrate family. The specific form of the sugar and the type of food it is packed within determines its digestion and effect on our bodies.

In the discussion of sugars and sweeteners, many people either cite the glycemic index or the amount of calories. I am not a fan of either, generally speaking, as the basic practice of eating should not involve tedious computations. We will never have to count calories if we are eating a whole, natural, plant-based diet, rich in vegetables and fruits. Such food offers high nutrient density in exchange for little calories and our bodies have the capacity to naturally regulate themselves with respect to optimal weight. Of course, we have to bring them back into their natural, regulatory balance first. Also, all calories are not equal, as we have already mentioned and will further discuss in Chapter 17. There is a big difference in fifty calories of white sugar versus fifty calories of raisins. This is of extreme importance, especially if trying to heal your body or lose weight.

When it comes to the glycemic index, some experts swear by it, while others feel it has too many flaws to be a credible tool of value. I tend to steer on the latter side of this matter. The glycemic index is a measure of the effects of carbohydrates on blood sugar. In the following examination of sweeteners, I will mention some glycemic index values for your interest, but please recognize that I do not steer my eating habits around the glycemic index, nor that of anyone else I teach or talk to. There are just too many other variables to consider, like what the food is eaten with and the health of your digestive system. Also, some healthy and wholesome foods are rated high (bad), while some unhealthy foods are rated low (good).

Refined Sugar

White sugar is a highly refined, acidic substance that has led to many health and weight problems, from increased infections to heart disease and nearly everything between. It has no nutritional value other than being a source of calories. Whether white or brown, refined sugar and any products containing it have no place in the diet and lifestyle of those of us who are taking accountability for our health, healing, and prevention. According to a USDA document that outlines dietary trends from 1970 to 2005, sugar consumption has increased by 19 percent since 1970, coming in at about 140 pounds of sugar per person, per year, 30 teaspoons of sugar per day!

The health problems associated with refined sugar run so deep and so much further than diabetes risk or weight gain. Refined sugar negatively influences every aspect of our physical, mental, and emotional health. It is one of the most destructive things to our immune system, making us more susceptible to all sorts of infections; from the common cold to rare skin infections. It is highly acid-forming, creating the perfect conditions for all sorts of vile pathogens, like candida and harmful bacteria, to thrive. It also wreaks havoc on our oral health, digestive health, bone health, and hormonal health.

Depression is one of the most debilitating health problems in our industrialized modern world today. Not only is it sharply on the rise, but according to the World Health Organization, it is also currently the fourth-leading contributor to the global burden of disease. Due to the fact that refined sugar interferes with proper serotonin production (our feel-good brain chemical), it has been linked to influencing the rates of depression. Refined sugar is highly addictive, as addictive as some drugs, and it is detrimental to proper emotional and mental balance, as well as energy levels. More information on the devastating effects of sugar can be found in Dr. Scott Olson's book, *Sugarettes*.

High Fructose Corn Syrup (HFCS)

As mentioned in Chapter 13, HFCS is one of the most toxic sweeteners we have. Corporations try to pass it as a "natural sweetener," since it comes from corn, but they fail to consider the chemical processing involved and the effects the products of this substance have on us. It is detrimental to our liver and overall health and directly correlated to current obesity in adults and children. A study published in the *American Journal of Clinical Nutrition* in 2004 demonstrated a major correlation of high fructose corn syrup and increased weight and outlined some other disturbing facts related to it. For example, consumption of HFCS increased more than 1000 percent between 1970 and 1990, and it now represents more than 40 percent of caloric sweeteners added to foods and beverages.[1] Since HFCS is only found in processed foods and drinks, simply avoiding those allows us to completely avoid this substance and the damage it can cause to our bodies.

Artificial Sweeteners

Artificial sweeteners such as saccharin, aspartame, or sucralose are another group of highly destructive sweeteners to our health. There are numerous health problems associated with each, and the symptoms or conditions they cause form a long list. Aspartame, which goes by several trade names and whose approval is considered the "the most contested in FDA history," is an excitotoxic neurotoxin and highly suspected carcinogen. It is mind-boggling how such substances are allowed to remain part of our food supply, though as we know, the practices of corporate politics leave a lot to be desired. As with HFCS, if we are serious about living in a state of optimal health for the best healing and prevention, we cannot consume processed foods that contain these ingredients or buy them to sweeten anything we eat. Make sure you also consider chewing gum or breath mints, as they are almost exclusively sweetened with artificial sweeteners. When it comes to gum, many people think they will not be affected because they do not swallow it, but chewing is part of digestion; during the chewing process, the various flavors, colors, chemicals, and artificial sweeteners are released and swallowed.

It is also prudent to mention here that many diabetics feel artificial sweeteners are their only choice when it comes to consuming sweeteners, that they have to select the alleged lesser of the evils. However, we know today that Type 2 diabetes, and certain Type 1 cases, can be reversed just by changing the food we eat. Look into the work of Drs. Gabriel Cousens or Joel Fuhrman to learn more about this, especially if you are currently dealing with diabetes. A diet based on processed food will not contribute to any healing or prevention; it only necessitates further chemical and pharmaceutical interventions. To attain healing, we must completely eliminate substances like artificial sweeteners from our diet and not rely on them under any circumstances.

Agave Nectar

Agave nectar or syrup seems natural and has been touted as a healthy sweetener in natural health circles for some time. However, as its popularity grew, we learned that it is, in fact, processed in ways that may not be favorable to our health. Also, it appears to contain an unhealthy amount and type of fructose; agave nectar or syrup is composed of anywhere from 60 to 90 percent fructose, depending on how it is processed, with the other part being glucose. It proudly claims to be a low-glycemic food, but this is only because of its high fructose content, which does not affect our blood-sugar levels like glucose. If one can find minimally processed, certified raw and organic versions of agave sweetener, it may be considered for occasional use, though I personally do not recommend it; there are other, similar sweeteners that are much better choices.

Stevia

Stevia is an herb in the chrysanthemum family, which grows as a wild, small shrub in parts of South America. Its incredible sweetness comes from specific compounds in its leaves. While it has been quite readily adopted by the natural health community, some precautions should be taken. Even though stevia has been used by indigenous South American peoples for centuries, many such plants must be treated more like medicine than food; recall our discussion about coffee. When it comes to our modern culture we tend to latch onto many things, be they natural plants, and use them recklessly. Modern research is inconclusive about stevia's full range of health pros and cons and stevia has experienced bans in several countries. I suspect that the safety and health effects of stevia are closely tied to the way it is processed and used, as is the case with most other sweeteners. Small, infrequent doses of wholesome, natural forms are probably just fine for us, whereas commercially processed ones, like Truvia, are not. If you are interested in using stevia and have any concerns, I invite you to explore this sweetener further.

Sugar Alcohols

Sugar alcohols, such as xylitol or sorbitol, are hydrogenated forms of carbohydrates. While considered safe, they have been known to cause various digestive and intestinal disturbances. This is mainly due to the fact that they are not easily absorbed or digested. They are lower in calories and sweetness, as compared to traditional sugar. As they are food derivatives rather than whole, real food, they are mainly found in processed food; thus, they should be easily avoidable. Certain natural foods contain some other forms of sugar alcohols that our bodies can process adequately, as they come as part of whole, natural food. They are not a common sweetener, but they have gained popularity in certain products. They do not appear to be detrimental, but since they are not exactly natural and wholesome either, they should be used with caution.

Coconut Sugar

With the surging popularity of coconut as a superfood in recent years, coconut products like coconut oil, butter, flour, and sugar have all gained positive status.

Coconut sugar is considered a natural sweetener, derived from the sap of the coconut palm tree flower buds, but it is not the same as palm sugar. The extraction process is similar to that of maple syrup; the sap must be collected and then heated to evaporate the water content. Advocates positively point out its nutritional potential and low glycemic index values. Its main composition is about 70 to 80 percent sucrose, which is broken down into glucose and fructose. It does have some nutrients, like potassium, iron, zinc, calcium, and some B vitamins, as well as some antioxidants. It also contains small amounts of fiber, inulin, amino acids, and fatty acids. Its sweetness is comparable to refined sugar, and it is a popular substitute where granulated sugar is called for. However, despite some of its positive attributes, we cannot forget that no isolated sugar should be used regularly or in large amounts.

Brown Rice Syrup

This is a rather foreign sweetener to most, but it can be a considerably good option where sweeteners are concerned. Brown rice syrup is made by culturing brown rice with enzymes. It is then cooked until the final syrup consistency is reached. Depending on how it is fermented, cultured, and heated, it may or may not be a truly raw product. It is not as sweet as honey or agave nectar, but it can be used widely to sweeten various foods.

What differentiates brown rice syrup from other sweeteners is its carbohydrate composition. Brown rice syrup consists of about 52 percent soluble complex carbohydrates, 45 percent maltose, and 3 percent glucose. The complex carbohydrates are mostly composed of *maltotriose*, three glucose molecules linked together. *Maltose* is composed of two glucose molecules linked together. For those concerned about fructose, this sweetener contains none. Glucose is easily used for fuel by our bodies, but too much at once causes blood-sugar imbalances and weight gain. The benefit of brown rice syrup is that the maltose needs to be broken down, which takes over an hour, as does the maltotriose, which can take two to three hours for full digestion. This considerably slows the amount of sugars going into the bloodstream and makes this sweetener not only a low-glycemic food but overall less threatening and more beneficial for our health in both the short and long term. Brown rice syrup also contains some beneficial minerals and other nutrients. If you ever choose to consume this sweetener, it is important, however, not to increase the quantities of it in an effort to match the sweetness of other sweeteners. Keep all isolated sweetener quantities to a minimum.

Despite all the positive news above, in recent years, concerns have surfaced about the quantities of arsenic found in rice products; specifically inorganic arsenic. This includes brown rice and brown rice syrup, even from organic sources. Governing bodies are still on the fence as to the safe amount and whether these small amounts have any negative impact on our long-term health. Many reputable rice companies, like Lundberg, are very transparent about their rice products and openly publish the results of their arsenic testing. While very low levels of arsenic naturally exist in many foods, it is good to be aware in order to make the most appropriate choices for your needs.

Maple Syrup

Maple syrup is a commonly considered choice when it comes to natural and healthy sweetener options. When it is of a high, pure quality, maple syrup can be considered a natural and even healthy sweetener. It provides some good nutritional density from minerals such as manganese, zinc, magnesium, calcium, iron, and potassium, some B vitamins, amino acids, organic acids, and antioxidants. Pure maple syrup is mostly sucrose, which breaks down into glucose and fructose. It has very little free glucose and fructose and is considered medium or low on the glycemic index. The production process uses heat to remove moisture from the maple sap, turning it into a syrup. The raw, watery sap is not considered maple syrup until the cooking process concentrates the sugars to a minimum of 66 percent of the product. If you are interested in using maple syrup in your diet, only choose pure, high-quality, hopefully local options that do not contain any preservatives or additives. Imitation maple-like syrups exist, often called "maple-flavored," but these are largely composed of high fructose corn syrup. Due to the high price tag of quality maple syrup, low-quality syrup is very common, and these may be heavily processed and diluted with other sweeteners, such as corn syrup. As with any sweetener, use sparingly.

Honey

Honey can be looked at from two interesting perspectives. On one hand, it is one of the oldest, most natural (purely nature-made), beneficial, and widely used sweeteners. On the other hand, its reputable heritage has many people relying on it too much, especially today, when most honey is heavily processed and devoid of its natural benefits. Honey may be included as part of an optimally healthy diet but only under three strict conditions. First, we must source pure, raw honey, not processed or pasteurized. Second, it must be consumed raw, meaning that we do not use it in any baking, cooking, or boiling-hot herbal tea. (Let your food or drink cool off a little before adding any in.) Third, we must use it very sparingly, not on a regular basis. If we consume conventional honey or bake with it, we are getting all the sugar without the nutrition and health benefits, which are destroyed with heat. Due to the denatured final product, refined, pasteurized, or heated honey is said to be no better than eating white table sugar. Imitation honey-like sweeteners also exist, so be very mindful about what you are consuming. For optimal healing and protective benefits, especially for allergies, asthma, and the immune system, honey should specifically come from local bee and flower sources.

Raw honey has been part of our human diet for thousands of years and carries many health and healing benefits. It is rich in vitamins, minerals, antioxidants, enzymes, phytonutrients, and other healing compounds and has even been called a superfood. It is about 18 percent water, 35 percent glucose, and 35 percent fructose, with small amounts of sucrose and maltose in composition. It is interesting to note that raw honey tends to be low on the glycemic index, while refined, pasteurized honey rates high. When it comes to honey, though, we have to take into account the modern collapsing of bee colonies around the world, resulting in sustainability challenges. Therefore, use it sparingly and responsibly for the sake of your health and the environment.

Dates

Although not a typical liquid or powdered sweetener, dates are, perhaps, the best way to incorporate a sweetener into our diet. Unlike all other isolated sugar sweeteners, dates are a whole, natural plant food that generally does not require any processing. They are also considered a raw food. They have been used throughout the Middle East as a valuable food source for thousands of years and have even been cited by a 2003 study published in the *International Journal of Food and Nutrition* as being "an almost ideal food, providing a wide range of essential nutrients and potential health benefits."[2] Not only are they alkaline-forming, but they are also a good source of fiber and at least six vitamins and fifteen minerals. They offer some protein, which shows an unusual composition of twenty-three amino acids.[2] Their sugar composition is a mixture of sucrose, glucose, and fructose. Nutrition facts vary based on the type of date, whether it is fresh or dried, and its ripeness. There are many varieties of dates, the three most common being deglet noor, honey, and medjool. All offer an incredibly sweet and delicious flavor, especially medjool, a prized delicacy. Dates can be used in a multitude of amazing, delicious, and healthy raw snacks and desserts.

Raisins

Raisins are also a whole, natural plant food and offer some valuable nutrients, including fiber. While not as nutritionally impressive as dates, they are a good choice, but we have to source out high-quality, organic varieties. Commonly available raisins often have added oils and preservatives and come from grapes that were sprayed with pesticides.

In the end, when it comes to sweeteners, common sense must prevail. Sweeteners, specifically isolated sugar sweeteners, regardless of how healthy-sounding, are not meant to be used in large quantities or on a regular basis. They should be used sparingly, as possible infrequent dietary additions. There are enough whole, sweet foods, like fresh or dried fruits, to add delicious sweetness to our diet. Our sugars should come in their most natural forms, with accompanying nutrients and fiber, and not as isolated nutrients. In this form, eating for optimal health can definitely include sweet flavors and many delicious meals. The key is to get all the processed food and processed sugars out of our diet first, detox our taste buds, then incorporate natural sweetener ideas sparingly, as appropriate to your needs.

Fermented Foods

While our goal is to keep our foods in their most natural and raw form, there is a form of food processing that is highly beneficial for our bodies and health. That process is fermentation, and it has been a valuable addition to human health for thousands of years. Fermented foods are some of the healthiest available, mostly due to the inclusion of healthy microorganisms, like various probiotics. Some of the health benefits for us include improved digestion, reduction of intestinal disorders, improved absorption, enhanced immunity, increased vitamin content, and enzyme composition. The beneficial microorganisms have been known to contain both antibiotic and anti-carcinogenic properties. However, it all depends on what we ferment and how.

Healthy fermented foods include vegetables, sauerkraut, kimchi, organic kefir, coconut milk, tempeh, miso, tamari, and shoyu. The last four are forms of fermented soy and can provide the safest and most nutritionally dense ways to enjoy the benefits of soy, as long as they are organic to avoid genetically modified soybeans. Tempeh is a nutritionally-dense, whole-food soy product that I highly recommend for its many health, flavor, and meal versatility benefits. It is completely different from tofu, which is a non-fermented and more nutritionally-stripped form of soy. Tamari and shoyu are nutritionally superior compared to common, processed soy sauce, but they are still extremely high in sodium, so should be used very sparingly, if at all. Numerous foods, especially vegetables, can be easily fermented at home and maintain their raw, whole-food qualities. The key to the healthiest fermentation is to use water and salt rather than vinegar, engaging in *lacto-fermentation*. Commercially fermented foods are seldom able to offer the same health benefits as those that have undergone lacto-fermentation. The majority of commercial sauerkraut or pickles are vinegar-based and contain various additives, sugars, and preservative agents that do not offer the same health benefits.

Similarly, despite all the marketing hype promoting commercial yogurt, it is a highly processed and unfavorable food for our health and weight, far from the health food it is often made out to be. Aside from the dairy problems themselves, most yogurt contains added sugars, artificial sweeteners, artificial flavors, colors, and preservatives. Additionally, commercial yogurt is both a direct and indirect source of genetically modified ingredients, including modified corn byproducts, GM lactic acid bacteria, genetically engineered bovine growth hormone, and GM food given to the animals. If you choose to eat any commercial yogurt, it should only be organic and plain, and you can add your own fruit to it as needed.

Fungi

Mushrooms are technically not vegetables and don't quite fall into any of the previous groups of food we have discussed. However, they must be an essential part of our discussion. Contrary to popular belief, mushrooms are nutritional powerhouses and optimally healthy food choices.

Mushrooms have been used as food and medicine for thousands of years, offering some of the most potent natural properties. They are outstanding for healthy weight maintenance and weight loss and provide many health benefits. They offer protection against infections and cancers, boost the immune system, and offer positive support for our digestive and heart health. They are rich sources of many vitamins, minerals, and antioxidants, including phytonutrients. We are just now grasping some of the more profound health benefits of mushrooms, which disciplines like Traditional Chinese Medicine have known for millennia. Mushrooms are 80 to 90 percent water and are very low in calories. They have very little sodium and fat, are a source of protein, and their dry weight is comprised of about 8 to 10 percent fiber. Not only do they offer an excellent profile of most vitamins and minerals, but mushrooms exposed to ultraviolet light are also reliable sources of Vitamin D.[3] Some, like common white button mushrooms, may even provide a reliable source of Vitamin B12.[4] When it comes to antioxidants, studies done on mushrooms have found them to possess outstanding antioxidant activity. This applies to various cultivated species,[5] but especially wild mushrooms.[6,7]

Enjoy an abundant variety of mushrooms regularly. Every type has something of benefit to offer, from the prized shiitake and maitake, right down to the common white button and crimini mushrooms. Wild mushrooms from local forests can also be used, but one must be a skilled mushroom expert to pick and safely use wild mushrooms. In terms of how to eat them, although there is still a lot that we do not know about mushrooms, the current consensus is that mushrooms should be cooked rather than consumed raw, as this makes them easier to digest. However, many people eat raw mushrooms routinely, and it may be the better way to go, as with our fruits and vegetables. Whether raw, sautéed, or stir-fried, it is easy to add mushrooms to soups, salads, and wraps or to use them in any appetizer or main vegetable-based dish. Explore the flavors and textures of the most common varieties found in grocery stores and markets: white button, crimini, portabella, oyster, enoki, chanterelle, morel, maitake, and shiitake mushrooms.

Another fungi that can be a beneficial part of an optimally healthy diet is nutritional yeast. It is an inactive yeast that comes in the form of small, yellow flakes and can be easily found at most bulk or health food stores. It has a strong flavor that some describe as nutty or cheesy. It is extremely high in B vitamins, with some brands even being a reliable source of Vitamin B12, and contains some minerals. It is rich in protein, low in fat and sodium, and free of dairy, gluten, and sugar. It can be eaten simply by sprinkling it on a salad or into a soup or on your main meal. Its flavor also makes it popular as an ingredient for cheese substitutes, as well as various dips, spreads, and sauces. It can mimic Parmesan cheese and when coupled with some other ingredients like raw cashews, it can create a delicious Alfredo-like sauce or creamy Caesar dressing. It can make all sorts of amazing wholesome, homemade goodies and has many people hooked on it. However, do keep in mind that despite its outstanding nutrition and versatility benefits, nutritional yeast is produced by humans and not nature; treat it more like a supplement than actual food.

Sea Vegetables

If you are fortunate enough to live near an ocean coast, you may have easy access to one of the healthiest foods on the planet: sea vegetables. We all know that vegetables are the optimal health foods, but we don't often think of the ocean as a place to source them. Sea vegetables include various seaweed and algae. The most common varieties are nori, dulse, wakame, kombu/kelp, sea lettuce, and arame. They have been part of Asian diets for centuries and are promoted for their many health and longevity benefits.

Sea vegetables are an excellent source of iodine. This is especially important, as more people are opting out of eating seafood due to the contamination of our oceans or as part of removing animal products from the diet. Plants are not as heavily affected as animals by pollution and toxic ocean contaminants. This is mainly due to the fact that they do not contain fat tissues, where most toxins are stored, and they are the lowest on the food chain. Sea vegetables are a great source of protein and vitamins and contain an abundance of minerals from the oceans. They also contain unique enzymes, antioxidants, and beneficial phytonutrients. Health benefits associated with sea vegetables are becoming increasingly known as we continue to unlock the secrets of these ocean plants. So far, research points to sea vegetables having benefits for all sorts of conditions. They can help regulate blood sugar and cholesterol, lower blood pressure and the risk of chronic diseases, including cancer, and they are antiviral and anti-inflammatory.

When purchased in their natural form, sea vegetables are pure, whole foods that retain their nutritional integrity and require no cooking. They are typically found in a dried form. A reputable company that provides high-quality options is Maine Coast Sea Vegetables. Avoid processed sea vegetables, which may be fried or have added oils, salt, and flavors. Sea vegetables can be eaten on their own as a snack or added to soups, salads, and various main dishes.

CHAPTER 15
Meal Ideas

While learning about your body, health, and nutrition is extremely valuable to help you implement positive lifestyle changes, little will happen unless we make eating for optimal health real and practical. Of course, what we consider practical can be very subjective, based on our personal perceptions. Some people find it practical to leave the house and drive to a nearby fast food restaurant to pick up dinner, while others find it practical to walk into their kitchen and prepare their own meal in the time that trip would take. Ultimately, what matters most is that you make your health and nutrition one of the main priorities in your life, if not your main consideration. Once this takes place, practical will take on a whole new meaning for you in terms of what makes most sense for maintaining your wellness at its best, healing present imbalances, and preventing future problems.

In this chapter, I will share with you some meal ideas to help you incorporate, on a practical level, all that has been presented thus far in terms of how and what to eat. This is not a typical recipe section. Many people continue to request that I publish a cookbook, and that may come at a future time, but primarily I prefer to empower and teach people how to work with their food naturally, creatively, and intuitively. No matter where you are or what you have available in terms of food ingredients, you should know how to nourish yourself optimally. Cookbooks and specific recipes may provide new meal ideas, but they may not be suitable for everyone's needs and preferences. The more you learn about your food, the different flavors, textures, and consistencies, the more resourceful you can be at putting together your meals.

When eating becomes real and wholesome, it can easily take on an effortless, creative flow. It also connects us mindfully to the food we eat, and how that food may impact our bodies. I personally almost never plan meals or fuss with measuring things to satisfy some specific recipe. I simply make sure my fridge and cupboards are always stocked with a wide variety of vegetables, fruits, nuts, seeds, beans, legumes, and whole, unprocessed grains, as well as some of the other optimally healthy food items mentioned in Chapter 14. From there, I gauge in the moment how much time I can spend preparing my meal. I follow through accordingly with a mix of food that suits those time constraints and available ingredients.

Some smart planning, however, should be taken into consideration based on your personal needs and lifestyle. If you tend to have busy weekdays, then prewashing and chopping your vegetables, as well as cooking a large batch of some grain, beans, and/or soup on the weekends will make meals easier to put together during the week. Many vegetables can be cut up ahead of time and stored in containers for faster use at meal time. We all have different life needs and circumstances. Some people are single, some have small kids, some can grow their own food, and some work nightshifts. We need to adapt our meal approach for optimal health accordingly, in order to make it work for us.

When it comes to special kitchen tools or appliances, I will provide a practical overview of these for you in Chapter 18. As with any other area of life, how well prepared you are will make all the difference in your success and satisfaction. The more you apply good organization habits and make effective use of your tools and time, the easier meal planning and preparation will become. For many of us, optimally healthy meal preparation will also require a shift in perspective. We need to see our food and its potential in a new light and the more we do, the more we will enjoy the process of nourishing ourselves. So, before we continue with practical meal ideas, let's review what the goal of our eating is. We want to make sure that our meals are based on:

1. **Real, whole, natural food**
2. **Plant food**
3. **Acid-alkaline balanced food**
4. **Raw food**
5. **Organic food**

Breakfast Meal Ideas

One of the main components of a diet that can easily meet all the criteria mentioned on the previous pages for optimal health, weight, healing, and prevention are vegetables—specifically dark, leafy, green ones. While most of us can imagine ways of incorporating those into our lunch and dinner, the task becomes a little more daunting when we consider greens for breakfast.

Whether we are interested in healing, prevention, or weight and health maintenance, we should all aim to have greens with most, if not all, meals. Recall the power of green foods from Chapter 3. A diet based on greens is especially important if we are trying to heal or balance our body after years of poor eating habits. At minimum, aim to have greens with at least two of your three main meals. Of course, the more closely you adhere to the five guidelines for eating and optimal foods discussed, the more powerful, effective, and rapid your health transformation will be. When we reduce the acidic load on the body, cleanse and detoxify, improve our intestinal health by supporting the healthy microflora, and lose excess weight, we reap the benefits of greater physical, mental, emotional, and energetic vitality. As your journey toward optimal health and nutrition continues, your dietary needs will continue to evolve naturally, and you will be able to better rely on your body's own feedback system as to what it needs to feel best at any given time.

Green Smoothies

The best way to incorporate greens for breakfast and start the day off with nutritional excellence are green smoothies. We will talk here about their practical nature and more about their characteristics in Chapter 19. They are super fast and easy to make, usually taking less than five minutes. This makes them a very practical breakfast option for everyone. Whether you are a single parent, a busy professional, or a student, they can be efficiently incorporated to meet everyone's needs. They can be consumed at home or easily taken with you on the road, whether you are heading to work or dropping kids off at school. Best of all, they are a delicious, light, yet filling, refreshing, and super-nutritious way to start your day.

You can have a simple green smoothie (fruits and veggies only) or a whole-meal green smoothie that includes other ingredients, like seeds. You can have a smaller portion (250 to 500 ml, or 8 to 16 ounces), or a larger portion (500 to 1000 ml, or 16 to 32 ounces). Where as a whole-meal green smoothie is satisfying on its own, a simple green smoothie can be combined with a bowl of oatmeal or some high-quality bread (such as Ezekiel sprouted whole-grain and legume bread) with nut butter.

Another positive attribute of green smoothies is that, as we play around and alternate the ingredients, we get to experience new flavors on a regular basis. Alternating the ingredients also ensures that you get a variety of different whole plant foods each day.

The table on the next page outlines some ingredients to get you started. You can mix and match different combinations and adjust quantities to meet your needs. The steps are super easy:

1. Pick the desired greens from the table, wash them, and place them into your blender. You can remove the thick inner stalk of leafy greens like kale, especially if you do not have a powerful blender. Start with anywhere from one to two large leaves or one cup or one handful of greens per serving and work your way up to more greens from there as your taste buds adjust.

2. Pick the desired fruits from the table, wash and/or peel them, and place them into your blender. A typical serving would include one to two whole fruits, roughly half-cup to two-cup equivalents. You can start with more fruit at the beginning and transition to less fruit and more greens as you progress.

3. Add in one to two servings of the healthy fat- and/or protein-rich ingredients. My personal recommendation is to go for about two tablespoons of the flax or chia seeds for the majority of your green smoothies. Beyond that, choose what may be most suitable for you and in what quantities, based on your health and lifestyle needs.

4. It is completely optional, but you may also wish to add a serving of one superfood (functional food) to your green smoothie. Each one has unique healing, protective, and restorative properties for specific needs. Research

any of the ones you are unfamiliar with to see how they may best suit your personal needs. They may be used daily for a particular span of time, periodically, or seasonally. Typically, anywhere from one teaspoon to one tablespoon is an adequate serving.

5.   Add some water, enough to cover a quarter or half of the ingredients in the blender. Add more water for a thinner consistency and less water for a thicker smoothie. Blend thoroughly, pour into a glass, and enjoy while fresh.

Non-dairy milks are possible but not recommended. They are processed food and should be used minimally, if at all. If you ever want to use a commercial, non-dairy milk, choose organic, unsweetened, unflavored varieties only. A homemade nut milk would be a much better choice. However, just adding some nuts into your smoothie can provide a richer, creamier smoothie in the most wholesome of ways.

Greens pick at least 1	Fruit pick 1 or 2	Healthy Fat and/or Protein-Rich Food pick 1 or 2	Superfood pick 1 (optional)
Kale	Banana	Hemp Seeds	Maca Powder
Collard Greens	Pineapple	Chia Seeds	Ashwagandha Powder
Swiss Chard	Berries	Flax Seeds	Chlorella Powder
Spinach	Mango	Other Seeds	Spirulina Powder
Bok Choy	Orange	Nut Butter	Cacao Powder
Dandelion	Red Grapes	Almonds	Camu Powder
Watercress	Apple	Other Nuts	Triphala Powder
Broccoli or Cabbage Leaves	Peach	Coconut (fresh or dried)	Gotu Kola Powder
Green Sprouts	Plum	Avocado	Goji Berries
Arugula	Apricot	Cooked Beans	Acai Berries

Ice cubes are optional, depending on whether you want your smoothie to have a chilled temperature or not, and they can be replaced by frozen fruit. While slightly chilled smoothies are okay, room temperature is best, and frigidly cold smoothies should be avoided.

As you become a seasoned smoothie drinker, you should naturally transition from less fruit to more greens and learn what works best for your taste preferences and health needs. If this is your first time trying a green smoothie, start with something simple, like the recipe below:

Simple Green Smoothie Starter Recipe

- 1 handful of spinach
- 1 banana
- 4 - 5 strawberries
- 2 tablespoons of chia or flax seeds (use ground if you don't have a high-powered blender)
- enough water to meet your consistency preference
- 1 to 2 ice cubes (optional)

I would like to make two final notes about green smoothies. First, the smoothness of the consistency will vary greatly, depending on the power of your blender. If you have a simple blender, expect to find pieces of the greens, fruits, and other ingredients or some grittiness. We will address the benefits of high-powered blenders in Chapter 18, which pulverize everything, for an extremely smooth consistency. Some people enjoy the bits of food in their smoothies, while others are put off by them, especially kids. Therefore, the ability of your blender to produce the right texture and consistency will make a big difference in the success and enjoyment of your smoothies.

Finally, green smoothies are not meant to be chugged or gulped down quickly. Think of them as you would a whole meal rather than a drink. To activate the proper digestion channels within your body, you should consume them mindfully, initiating a chewing-like movement with each mouthful. This is where thicker smoothies help, as they naturally make you want to chew. Thicker smoothies also allow us to consume more nutrients before getting full, due to the smaller volume of the final product, as opposed to it having a higher water volume. The latter, though, may be helpful if you are trying to lose weight.

Fruit & Vegetable Salad

Another great way to start the day is with a side or whole-meal fruit and/or vegetable salad. Actually, when it comes to breakfast, we need to break out of the mold that certain foods are breakfast foods, while others aren't. We can easily enjoy a plant-based salad anytime of the day and this includes breakfast. Your breakfast salad can include traditional fruits, or focus on vegetable fruits like cucumbers, tomatoes, and avocados.

Fruit and vegetable salads also provide a great way to start the day with some leafy greens. Perhaps green smoothies just aren't your thing, or you want to change things up for the weekend breakfast. Either way, salads can provide a nutritionally dense and filling start to your day. Enjoy experimenting with all sorts of leafy greens, fruit, and vegetable combinations. To make your salad a whole-meal option, include various nuts, seeds, or beans. You can also add unique spices and flavors with ingredients like nutritional yeast or put your favorite homemade dressing added on top. For more salad ideas, refer to the "Lunch & Dinner Meal Ideas" section that follows.

Breakfast Grains

For some breakfasts, you can enjoy a whole, unprocessed grain. This can include a bowl of steel-cut oats, teff, kamut, or quinoa. remember to make it a *real* grain, as opposed to a refined grain product. Any boxed cereals, no matter how healthy they claim to be, should be avoided. When adding milk to boxed cereal, even non-dairy varieties, we consume a processed-food breakfast and a fully acid-forming one. Cooking times for real, whole grains vary from two minutes (oat bran) to twenty-five minutes (millet), making them ideal to suit almost anyone's schedule. You might recall that all grains can be made easier to digest and nutritionally more robust by soaking them, which can easily be done overnight and decreases their cooking time. They are wonderful served warm with fresh or dried fruit, some nuts or seeds, and spices.

You can also include minimally processed grains in the form of high-quality bread, like Ezekiel, which, as we learned in Chapter 10, is made from whole, sprouted grains and legumes. A slice or two of Ezekiel bread or an Ezekiel wrap can be accompanied by homemade nut or seed butters, or minimally processed, raw and organic, store-bought versions. Alternatively, you can use some mashed avocado or a bean spread, like hummus to top your bread or wrap. Your grain bowl or bread grain can be accompanied by a simple green smoothie or salad to add some fruits and leafy greens to your meal.

Other Breakfast Ideas

Some mornings, you may desire something entirely different for breakfast. Also, if you need to transition from refined carbohydrate breakfasts that are full of refined sugars and other additives you may find it difficult to switch over to a breakfast salad or green smoothie. Whether you need something to ease your transition or just for the odd change-it-up-a-bit occasion, there are many ways to turn unhealthy options into more wholesome food choices. An example are crepes, pancakes, muffins, or granola bars. If and when these items are made at home from the most wholesome, organic, plant ingredients, they can be a nutritious addition to the diet. However, we must remember that subjecting our food to high or prolonged temperatures is not ideal. Similarly, any use of flour means we are not using grains in their most optimal way. Thus, it is essential that these foods are used infrequently, if at all, or merely as transition items as you take steps to optimize your diet.

If you must use flour, always choose whole and organic and preferably not wheat flour. For example, try spelt flour. If you are trying to avoid gluten, try brown rice flour, chickpea flour, or gluten-free flour options from companies like Bob's Red Mill. Remember that no flour is an optimally healthy food source, so flour-based products should be the exception, not the norm in your diet. When making crepes or pancakes, be mindful not to use any unhealthy oils or sugars. Below is an example of a simple crepe recipe, one of the healthiest possible:

Vegan, Gluten-Free Chia Crepes

- 1 cup Bob's Red Mill All-Purpose, Gluten-Free Baking Flour
- 1 tbsp. Organic Chia Seeds (use ground, if not using high-powered blender)
- 1 tbsp. Organic, Virgin Coconut Oil
- 1 cup Organic Non-dairy Milk (homemade or least processed)
- ½ cup Water

Blend all ingredients together. Pour batter evenly into an appropriate, thoroughly heated pan and cook like traditional crepes, a few minutes on each side. This recipe will yield roughly four ten-inch crepes. Serve with fresh fruit and a nut butter for a sweet version or with leafy greens, diced veggies, and hummus for a more savory flavor. You can check out more of my healthy meal ideas and recipes on www.EvolvingWellness.com

For optimal health and weight, avoid these common breakfast foods: bacon, sausage, fried eggs, fried potatoes, cheese, cow's milk, boxed cereals, cold cuts, white or brown wheat bread, conventional pancakes, waffles, muffins, pastries, doughnuts, granola bars, juice, and coffee.

Lunch & Dinner Meal Ideas

When it comes to lunch and dinner, you really do not need to differentiate between the two, aside from practical considerations. We have all become creatures of habit and often adhere to the illusory societal norms, believing that certain foods or meals are only for breakfast, lunch, or dinner. There is no reason to put such limitations upon ourselves or our food. Generally speaking, though, we should avoid eating late or consuming large, heavy meals for dinner. We should eat real, whole food at all meals and in appropriate portions to make us feel satisfied but not full. Other than that, listen to your body and respect its communication signals.

It is also important to avoid skipping meals. Too many people revolve their life around their work at the expense of their health, not to mention other things. A point of starvation or extreme fatigue is reached and the most common food choice at that point is whatever is the quickest, whether that be a chocolate bar or a fast-food combo. This is not how optimal health or weight is created; we must make our food and meal times a priority. This means taking the necessary time to plan ahead and consciously consume food in a relaxed fashion. Skipping meals or eating on the go or while stressed and hurried does a number on our digestion and metabolism and ultimately does not work to support the body, a healthy weight, or overall health. Just the act of chewing has enough power to increase or decrease the efficiency with which we will break down, properly digest, and assimilate a meal. When you make time for your meals, you make time for your health. Also, whether we are dealing with weight challenges or not, all of us can benefit from regular eating intervals to optimize our metabolism, blood-sugar balance, and overall body functions.

Soups

One of the easiest and most neglected meals is good, old-fashioned soup. Within this group, we include stew and chili. Today, most people buy soup in a can, a carton, or from a restaurant. If soup is made at home, it is almost always based on processed stock, which is typically loaded with sodium and many other unhealthy ingredients. Instead, we can make wholesome, natural, nutrient-dense soups at home that are easy, fast, and very rewarding for our health. In this way, we have full control over the amount and quality of the ingredients in our soups. We simply need to release two limiting beliefs that many of us hold when it comes to homemade soups. The first is that a good soup is hard to make or takes a long time. The second is that soups require some kind of stock. The truth is that soups can be very easy and fast to make and absolutely do not require any stock. It all depends on how we work with our base ingredients, herbs, and spices.

The following table shows some examples and ideas to help get you started. Each soup listed here is made with whole, natural ingredients, and none use any animal or vegetable stock or bouillon cubes, as these products are very high in sodium and are processed foods. These healthy soups are simply based on water. The trick to any great homemade soup is to let the natural bean and vegetable flavors penetrate through, while enhancing the overall flavor with a variety of herbs and spices.

Lentil Soups	Bean Soups	Squash Soups	Vegetable Soups
• Rinse lentils thoroughly and cook in plenty of water on low heat. • Cool as needed and purée in blender, adding more water if necessary.	• Use a dry bean soup mix or make your own dry bean mix. • Use 4-6 cups of water for every 1 cup of dry mix. • Add more water if adding some of the vegetables below.	• Cut a squash in half and remove the seeds. Steam the squash on low heat, in a base of water. • Let cool, remove skin, and purée in blender with enough water.	• Cook a mix of diced, fresh vegetables on low heat, in enough water. • Hard vegetables need more time to cook than soft ones, so add to pot accordingly.

POSSIBLE ADD-INS:			
Carrots	Carrots	Lentils or Beans	Potato or Yam
Tomatoes	Cauliflower	Whole Grains	Carrots
Bell Peppers	Broccoli	Coconut Oil	Beets
Mushrooms	Celery	Tomatoes	Celery
Sea Vegetables	Sea Vegetables	Sea Vegetables	Cauliflower

POSSIBLE FLAVOR-ENHANCING IDEAS:			
Herbs: fresh or dried cilantro, oregano, etc.	**Herbs:** fresh or dried basil, oregano, etc.	**Herbs:** fresh or dried basil, thyme, mint, etc.	**Herbs:** fresh or dried: basil, dill, oregano, etc.
Spices: cayenne, ginger, coriander, masala, turmeric, etc.	**Spices:** cayenne, black pepper, ginger, cumin, etc.	**Spices:** ginger, pepper, cinnamon, turmeric, etc.	**Spices:** turmeric, black pepper, ginger, cumin, etc.

Salt (Himalayan or Unrefined Sea Salt)

Lemon Juice (freshly squeezed) or some **Apple Cider Vinegar**
(add to soup after it is finished cooking)

Onion and garlic can transform any meal, including soups. Experiment with freshly chopped or dry, powdered versions. Go gentle on the garlic, as too much can result in a bitter or very sharp, spicy flavor.

Experiment with a dash of herbs, spices, and/or salt, stir well, and add in more of the flavor-enhancing herbs and spices, based on your taste preference. These can be added at the start, in the middle, or at the end of cooking. Explore to learn what works for you and your particular soup. Refer to the "Herbs & Spices" section in Chapter 14 for more tips.

Even though soups are usually cooked, as long as we don't overcook our ingredients, we can still take advantage of the many benefits. Also, any water-soluble nutrients that leach out of the ingredients will still be present in the soup liquid (broth) we consume. Soups can easily include all the macro- and micronutrients, which makes them a great whole-meal option. They tend to be low in calories, high in nutrients, and offer a satisfying meal for the whole family. They can be enjoyed warm, made with steamed or gently cooked ingredients, and this is especially useful during the cold months. They can also be enjoyed cool, made from fully raw or gently steamed ingredients, which is useful during the hot months. You can enjoy a variety of textures and consistencies as well, from thick and chunky to light and puréed versions. They can serve as a very practical meal, since you can make a large pot of a soup and use it for several of your lunch or dinner meals in the days that follow.

Salads

A popular and simple meal that can easily satisfy our criteria for healing and prevention comes in the form of salads. In fact, we should always aim to consume a large, whole-meal salad once a day. These are not the typical salad, a few pieces of iceberg lettuce and tomato slices with a bottled salad dressing. These are also not salads loaded with potatoes and mayonnaise. Rather, whole-meal, healthy salads are based on a variety of fresh, natural, whole-food ingredients and cover the full range of macro- and micronutrients. They can be lower or higher in calories, depending on your needs, but they are always nutrient dense and filling. Normally, the more vibrantly or diversely colorful your salad is, the more benefits it offers for your health. Be liberal with your vegetables, adding in lots of variety, and be sure to eat a large enough portion, treating it like a main meal and not a side dish.

The following table outlines some possible combinations. Enjoy mixing and matching the numerous options for tasty, wholesome salads. The steps are very straightforward:

1. Pick the desired greens from the table, wash them, chop or shred as needed, and place them into your bowl. You can remove the thick inner stalk of leafy greens like kale.

2. Pick the desired vegetables, wash and/or peel as needed, chop or dice, and place them into your bowl.

3. Add in one to two ingredients from the healthy fat- and/or protein-rich options. My personal recommendation is to go for about four to six tablespoons of a cooked bean or lentil for the majority of your salads. Beyond that, choose what may be most suitable for you and in what quantities, based on your health and lifestyle needs.

4. Add in a flavor-enhancing combination of your choice from the toppings category. You can also create various homemade dressings, such as the example I share below, to use on your salads.

Greens Pick at least 1	Vegetables Pick 2 to 3	Protein and/or Fat-Rich Food Pick 1 to 2	Toppings Pick several
Romaine Lettuce	Tomato	Hemp Seeds	Lemon Juice
Baby Greens	Broccoli	Ground Chia Seeds	Lime Juice
Spinach	Cauliflower	Ground Flax Seeds	Herbs
Arugula	Radish	Organic Tempeh	Spices
Green or Red Leaf Lettuce	Bell Peppers	Cooked or Sprouted Lentils	Raw Apple Cider Vinegar
Kale	Cucumber	Cooked or Sprouted Beans	Nutritional Yeast
Swiss Chard	Carrots	Nuts	Garlic
Cabbage	Zucchini	Avocado	Onion
Wild Leafy Greens	Peas	Olives	Ginger

Numerous salad dressings can easily be made in a vinaigrette or creamy form, adding robust, flavorful, whole-food, natural, nutrient-dense ingredients to your salads. Experiment with ginger, fresh-squeezed orange or lime juice, raspberries, apple cider vinegar, balsamic vinegar, poppy seeds, tahini, nutritional yeast, cashews, sunflower seeds, etc.

Homemade Herbed Salad Dressing Recipe

Mix the ingredients below in a blender or small dish, then pour over salad. This amount will typically satisfy two whole-meal salads. Double or triple the ingredients if you need to make enough for a larger group or for later use; it will keep well in the refrigerator for up to two weeks.

- **Garlic:** 1 clove (mince, if not using a blender)
- **Lemon Juice:** 1 large, fresh lemon, squeezed
- **Olive, Flax, or Hemp Oil:** 1to 2 tbsp. (optional)
- **Salt:** dash of Himalayan or Unrefined Sea Salt
- **Pepper:** dash of black pepper, cayenne pepper, or both
- **Spices:** ¼ to ½ tsp of ground cumin
- **Herbs:** some dried basil and/or oregano and/or rosemary

Wraps & Sandwiches

Whether for lunch, dinner, or even breakfast, wraps and sandwiches make an easy, quick, satisfying meal idea. They are especially easy to take with you to work or for your children to carry to school. They can include a wide variety of macro- and micronutrients and meet our optimal health and nutrition needs.

The most important thing to keep in mind about wraps and sandwiches is that we mustn't base our diet on them, nor should we use them in ways that will work against us rather than for our health. You may recall from Chapter 10 that neither refined bread products nor flour-based products are optimally healthy. For grains to work beneficially for us, they have to be consumed with alkaline-rich foods and should be whole, soaked, sprouted, or fermented. This is why natural, high-quality Ezekiel bread or sourdough products can be our only considerations here for optimal health.

1. Pick a low-sodium, minimally processed, whole-grain, flourless Ezekiel or whole-grain sourdough bread, or tortilla. (Remember to check the ingredients for any hidden sugars, white or non-whole flours, unhealthy fats, additives, and preservatives.)

2. Use a homemade or minimally processed bean, lentil, nut, or seed spread or butter, such as hummus, tahini, or sunflower butter. Alternately, or in addition to, you can use natural mustard or a mashed avocado as a spread. Avoid all margarine, butter, mayonnaise, and commercial condiments.

3. Add into the wrap or sandwich a leafy green and two to three raw or lightly cooked vegetables; include more on the side.

4. Add in other food items: sprouts, mushrooms, tempeh, sea vegetables, etc.

5. Enhance your wrap or sandwich with herbs and spices, as may be desired.

Stir-Fried, Sautéed, & Steamed Veggie Mixes

Various combinations of whole, natural, nutritionally dense meals for optimal health can also easily come in the form of a stir-fry or from steamed or sautéed ingredients. The key is simply to lightly cook the food for a short period of time rather than applying excessive or prolonged heat. Even though these tend to be healthier heat-processing options than roasting, grilling, or frying, overcooking our food can still work against us. There are two clues to let you know if your food is overcooked: color and texture. When greens are steamed, they typically become more deep, vibrant green. This is okay, but we need to avoid discoloration that causes the greens to become olive-green or even brownish. This is a clue that they have lost many of their valuable nutrients. Also avoid browning your food. As for texture, vegetables should be crisp or mildly hard rather than soft or mushy for best nutrient integrity and palatability.

Here are the basic steps to get you started. Refer to the chart on the following page for ingredient ideas.

1. In a large pan or skillet, heat a small amount of water, about one to two tablespoons. You can also use nothing, which is especially good if you are starting out with mushrooms or wet vegetables, such as zucchini. These will release a lot of their own juices, specifically if cooking while covered. If you choose to use oil, only consider virgin, coconut oil as we discussed in Chapter 14.

2. Add some minced garlic and/or onion (optional).

3. Add vegetables and mushrooms, giving them enough time to gently soften; typically five to fifteen minutes. Start with the mushrooms and your hardest vegetables like cauliflower or carrots. Your leafy greens must be last, left only to steam on top of the mix for the final couple of minutes.

4. Sprinkle in some of your favorite herbs, spices, and other possible additions. (See table below for ideas.) You can also create various whole-food sauces and creamy curries to add to your mix.

5. Stir occasionally and cook on low to medium heat, covered for a steamed mix or uncovered for a stir-fry. Normally, this will take less than fifteen minutes.

6. Serve with a side of one, possibly two, of the following: cooked, steamed, or sprouted beans or legumes; whole, unprocessed gains, such as brown rice, buckwheat, or quinoa; potatoes or yams; organic tempeh or tofu; deep-, cold-water fish or an organic meat.

Just like you choose healthy foods, choose healthy cookware. Nonstick pans, especially Teflon-based, have been linked to numerous health problems. We will cover this further in Chapter 18.

Greens Pick at least 1	Vegetables Pick 2 to 4	Mushrooms Pick 1 or more	Additions Pick several
Kale	Eggplant	Portabella	Herbs
Collard Greens	Zucchini	Crimini	Spices
Swiss Chard	Bell Peppers	White Button	Garlic
Spinach	Cauliflower	Shiitake	Onion
Cabbage	Broccoli	Oyster	Seeds
Rapini	Asparagus	Enoki	Nuts
Bok Choy	Tomatoes	Maitake	Sea Vegetables
Dandelion	Brussels Sprouts	Chanterelle	Lemon/Lime Juice
Arugula	Squash	Morel	Tamari/Shoyu Sauce

Dessert & Snack Ideas

Optimal health does not mean you must give up sweet treats. Countless dessert and snack ideas can be easily made for regular consumption and special occasions alike. The best, healthiest, easiest desserts and snacks come from food in its most pure, natural forms. These types of snacks and desserts revolve mainly around raw or dried fruits and nuts or seeds. To diversify the flavors and textures, it all comes down to how we mix those fruits, nuts, and seeds. A wealth of whole-food, plant-based, raw desserts exists and these are a sensation for our taste buds and nutritionally dense for our health. They can take on various flavors, sweetness, textures, and visual appeal. Best of all, most of them do not depend on or require any isolated sweeteners.

I will provide two versatile dessert and snack ideas to get you started. Where you go from there will depend on your personal needs, preferences, and creativity. Numerous whole-food, plant-based, raw, natural dessert and snack recipes can be found online, including my sites: www.EvolvingWellness.com for text recipes and www.Healthytarian.com for video recipes. Today, we can enjoy chocolate sauces, spreads, and fudge; raw brownies, cookies, pies, and cakes;

granola and energy bars; and more in the most optimally healthy of ways! These require no baking, and all of them can be made without refined sugars, flours, unhealthy fats, animal products, additives, or preservatives.

> Do not consume desserts directly after meals. It is best to use desserts as snacks between meals. This is optimal for our digestion, health, and weight.

The Optimal Nut & Fruit Snack Mix

Bars, squares, balls, cupcakes, cake crusts, bases, layers, and even cookie-cutter shapes can be easily made with two simple ingredients: nuts (or seeds) and a dried fruit. In terms of quantity, always use more nuts than fruit. The quantity will depend on what kind of texture and taste you desire. For coarser, crumblier mixtures to make into bars, crusts, or crumble toppings, use more nuts. For smoother, stickier textures, use closer to a one:one nut:dry fruit ratio. It is important to note that this mixture cannot be ruined, so go ahead and have fun with it! Get creative and see what consistency and flavor combinations you most enjoy.

Simply add the nuts (or seeds) and dried fruit into a food processor and blend until you have a sticky or crumbly mixture. Typically, about one and a half cups of nuts is combined with one cup of dried fruit to make sixteen squares in an eight-inch square dish or about twenty-four balls. The texture will depend on the power of your machine, the type of dried fruit and nuts or seeds used, the time of processing, whether the nuts have been soaked, other ingredients present, etc. Shorter processing time results in a more crumbly mixture, while a longer processing time results in a more sticky mixture.

The mix can be shaped or pressed into any shape or container with one's fingers or an appropriate kitchen tool. If the final product is a ball, it can be coated by rolling each one in cacao powder or shredded coconut for easier handling and enhanced visual appeal. If you have kids, you can roll out the mix and let them use cookie cutters to make different shapes.

Start in an easy way by choosing one nut and one dried fruit (see table) to gain an understanding of how the base ingredients will act and taste. Then get creative and have fun with new combinations. Your future creations can include some of the flavorings and additions; you literally have hundreds of possible combinations are your fingertips!

Nut or Seed Pick 1	Dried Fruit Pick 1	Flavorings Optional	Additions Optional
Almonds	Medjool Dates	Vanilla (bean or extract)	Raw Cacao Powder
Cashews	Honey Dates	Mint (fresh or extract)	Raw Cacao Nibs
Walnuts	Deglet Noor Dates	Pure Almond Extract	Shredded Coconut
Hazelnuts	Dried Figs	Cinnamon	Coconut Butter
Brazil Nuts	Goji Berries	Cardamom	Carob Powder
Pecans	Raisins (oil and preservative-free)	Nutmeg	Camu Powder
Macadamia Nuts	Apricots (sulfur-free)	Lemon (fresh juice or zest)	Spirulina Powder
Sunflower Seeds	Prunes (oil and preservative-free)	Orange (fresh juice or zest)	Maca Powder
Hemp Seeds	Golden/Inca Berries	Lime (fresh juice or zest)	Lucuma Powder
Pumpkin Seeds	Dried Cranberries (sugar and oil-free)	Ginger	Acai Powder
Sesame Seeds	Dried Blueberries (sugar and oil-free)	Organic Coffee Bean Granules	Maqui Powder

The Optimal miMIC Cake Mix

This is another highly versatile recipe that can be catered to meet your taste and texture preferences. Since it mimics a mousse cake, ice cream cake, and cheesecake, I call it "miMIC cake." I will provide you with some basic measurements and general guidelines. Once you get the hang of it, you will find that it is easy to play with and make all sorts of variations. The following serving is meant for an eight- to ten-inch round cake or pie dish.

Crust

- 1 to 1 ½ cup raw macadamia nuts or almonds (presoaked for 4-8 hours)
- 6 larger to 8 smaller medjool dates (pits removed)
- Finely shredded natural coconut flakes (optional)

Crust Instructions

1. Sprinkle some of the coconut in the dish, lightly dusting the bottom of the dish. This is completely optional, and the cake will still come out of the dish easily without the coconut.

2. Place the nuts and dates in a food processor and blend until the mixture is relatively smooth and sticky.

3. Transfer the mixture into the dish, spread evenly, and using your fingers press, making a crust that covers the base and sides evenly.

Filling

- 1 to 1 ½ cup raw cashew nuts (presoaked in water for 4 hours)
- 2 to 3 tbsp. virgin coconut oil or coconut butter
- ¼ to ½ cup of cold water
- **Flavor combinations:** 1 tsp. of natural vanilla or mint; juice of 1 fresh lime or lemon; 1 ripe banana or mango; or 2 tbsp. of raw cacao or carob powder (pick one or two of these per cake)
- **Optional:** depending on your taste preference and whether or not you are using any fresh fruit, if you are using the raw cacao, you may need 1 or 2 tbsp. of maple syrup or raw honey

Filling Instructions

1. Place all the ingredients in a food processor and blend until mixture is smooth and creamy.

2. Taste the mixture to see if you need to add anything else. Be prepared: The crust will be sweet enough to balance out the normally less sweet filling.

3. More or less water can be added, depending on how thick you want the filling to be. Filling should flow like typical batter but not be runny. More water will be better for mousse-like cake, and less water will be better for cheesecake- or ice-cream-like cake.

4. Pour filling into dish with the prepared crust, smoothing out the top with a spatula.

5. Place in the refrigerator or freezer to chill sufficiently and serve, normally allowing two hours for the cake to set. Cake should harden enough to be cut smoothly and maintain its shape. Storing the cake in the freezer makes an ice cream-like cake.

6. Cake should be stored in either the fridge or freezer at all times.

> As you experiment with different options, replace the cashews with fresh fruit and the coconut oil with coconut butter for a lighter cake that is lower in fat and calories. Good fresh fruit options include bananas, strawberries, blueberries, raspberries, and mango.

Whatever combination you choose to enjoy from the above mentioned snack choices, do stay mindful of your portion sizes and serving amounts. Since these types of snacks and desserts are based on nuts and seeds they are not only nutrient-rich but also calorie-rich. Assuming one miMIC cake yields eight slices and one typical Fruit & Nut Mix yields sixteen squares in an eight-inch dish or 24 balls, a serving of each would be as follows: one slice, one square, or two balls. Young, growing children or active individuals can increase the servings or portion sizes as appropriate for their needs.

Other Snack/Dessert Ideas

1. **Fresh Fruit Salad.** Any single fruit or combination of fresh fruits, chopped or diced and mixed together. Possible toppings include raw cacao nibs, nuts, seeds, raw cacao sauce, shredded coconut, etc.

2. **Raw Nuts.** A handful of raw nuts, preferably soaked, can be eaten as a quick and simple snack.

3. **Ice Fruit Cream.** If you have a high-powered blender, like a Vitamix, as we will discuss in Chapter 18, simply put some frozen fruit in and blend until smooth but firm. Mixture will resemble ice cream. You can add nut butter or coconut butter for a richer, creamier consistency. Other possible additions include raw cacao powder for chocolate ice cream. You can also use soaked cashews, frozen banana, and pure vanilla extract for a rich, creamy vanilla ice cream.

4. **Nut or Seed Milk Shakes.** You can make your own homemade nut or seed milk easily, depending on the tools you have. Some juicers can extract the milk of soaked nuts, and high-powered blenders can turn whole nuts into a smooth milk or milk shake. The blended milk can then be strained through a cloth bag to produce a silky milk. You can also add fruit, raw cacao powder, and ice cubes to the nut or seed mixture to make all sorts of milkshake combinations.

5. **Dried Fruits.** Dates, prunes, apricots, figs, or other dried fruits that have no added sugars, oils, or preservatives can be used. You can also finely slice your own fruits and dry them in a dehydrator, or sun dry them on hot, sunny days to make your own dehydrated fruit. Sun-dried strawberries, thinly sliced, are like candy!

6. **Veggie Sticks or Slices.** Fresh vegetable sticks or slices (celery, carrots, kohlrabi, radish, etc.) make great, optimally healthy, versatile snacks. These can be served with a homemade dip, like hummus or nut butter.

7. **Vegetable Chips.** Finely sliced or shredded root vegetables like beets work well, as do greens like kale. Shredded or sliced veggies can be seasoned with herbs and salted for flavor, then dried in the sun or a dehydrator.

8. **Grainless Crackers.** If you have a dehydrator, you can make all sorts of raw, grainless crackers using various vegetable, seed, herb, and spice combinations. These are great tasting and satisfying on their own or with homemade bean spreads and dips, like hummus.

PART 3

Beyond Food

"It's up to you today to start making healthy choices. Not choices that are just healthy for your body, but healthy for your mind."

— Dr. Steve Maraboli

CHAPTER 16
Supplements

An exploration of nutrition today would be incomplete without covering the topic of supplements and the role they play in our diet and health. Supplements represent one of the fastest-growing industries and one of the largest. *Nutraceuticals World* reported that global dietary supplement sales were estimated at $187 billion in 2008 and are projected to reach $204.8 billion by 2017. Supplements typically include vitamins and minerals, herbs, phytonutrients, homeopathics, and many other dietary supplements like fish oils. The current supplement trends and statistics present some interesting findings for us to consider. Let's examine some of these before we look at what may help us on our journey of healing and prevention and what may not.

A large part of the population has come to depend heavily on supplement use. According to the Center for Disease Control and Prevention, in the early 2000s, over 50 percent of U.S. adults were using supplements. The 2013 *Council for Responsible Nutrition* consumer survey reported that 68 percent of U.S. consumers are now using dietary supplements. However, a good portion of the population also opposes supplement use. In the October 2013 issue of *Nutraceuticals World*, data showed that one-third (34 percent) of adults are now confident that the foods they eat satisfy all their nutritional requirements.[1]

When one examines this market and the products within it via thorough holistic and scientific analysis, it becomes obvious that a large portion of the supplements created, purchased, and used are unnecessary. Some provide no positive health effects, and some actually negatively impact our health. Others are simply a waste of financial and environmental resources. Although it may seem as if the producers have good intentions, offering a natural and holistic dietary or healing aid, supplements are products, and they do have profit at their foundation. This is simply not something we can overlook.

The good news is that more of us are becoming increasingly critical and discerning consumers who are not so easily lured by the cleverly marketed multivitamin formula or cheapest generic herb. We are beginning to ask questions and seek satisfactory answers before we invest our money or put our health at risk. People are starting to see a pill for just what it is: a pill, not some equivalent or superior product to whole, natural food. An increasing number of individuals are raising concerns about supplements: How much is actually absorbed by our bodies? What is the quality, potency, or purity of the product? To be wise consumers, we must read all of the ingredients in our foods and supplements. When we do, we become more empowered to seek products that do not include any colors, flavors, preservatives, or other questionable fillers and additives. We should demand the purest, most effective products, but at this point in the supplement market, these are few and far between.

My personal stance on supplements and my recommendation for you is to always seek all you need from your food first. No pill or powder will ever replace whole, natural, plant food of the highest quality. Nevertheless, there are many variables to consider and it would be presumptuous to simply categorize supplements as good or bad. We have to consider our present health, dietary and lifestyle habits, the type of product, its quality, and its intended use if we are to effectively determine whether it may be of help, no use, or harm. Either way, our primary goal should always be nutritional excellence. If there is a substance that can help us further, above and beyond nutritional excellence, it may definitely be worthy of consideration.

Multivitamins

Multivitamins are among the most popular and widely used supplements today. According to a report from the National Center for Health Statistics from 2011, multivitamins are the most commonly used dietary supplement, with approximately 40 percent of men and women reporting use from 2003 to 2006.[2] The 2013 Council for Responsible Nutrition consumer survey confirms that multivitamins are still the most commonly used supplement, now estimated to be taken by 52 percent of U.S. adults. Parents give multivitamins to their children from a young age, paving the road for regular lifetime use. Adults of all ages rely on multivitamins as a type of insurance policy, hoping it will trump a poor or questionable diet. Many live in the false belief that multivitamins will improve their health and help protect them from various acute and chronic conditions. Others believe that taking a multivitamin is part of a healthy lifestyle. The reasons for use are many; unfortunately, the actual benefits are few, as modern health statistics and research have validated. Many experts agree that convincing scientific evidence of any true health benefit from multivitamin use is lacking. Additionally, doctors and health professionals are not the most likely reason behind a consumer's choice to use multivitamins; rather, it stems from persuasive marketing.

Due to my deep understanding of the power of whole, natural plant food, my personal opinion about multivitamins does not line up in their favor. Too many people falsely rely on multivitamins rather than changing their diet to be based on whole, natural, nutrient-rich food. Too many swallow pills simply out of habit, without understanding how they work. There is no doubt that some fear and insecurity has been instilled in the public by various voices who claim that, despite our best dietary efforts today, we cannot possibly glean enough vitamins and minerals for our needs from our food. However, when we examine where these claims are coming from on a deeper level, they appear to stem from one of two areas.

First, some groups or experts lower the bar tremendously when it comes to what we are capable of, not giving the majority of people credit for having the ability to eat a high-quality diet. This approach does not resonate with me, as it is extremely disempowering. I prefer to raise the bar to inspire and motivate people, to equip them with all the right tools, resources, and support to know that they can do it and consume a nutritionally-rich diet. Second, many of these claims are based on meeting the current RDA (recommended dietary allowance, also known as RDI or DRI) for vitamin and mineral intake, even though these numbers are controversial, commonly disputed, and quite artificial in their nature. What we are told we need in terms of any macro- or micronutrients are in no way universal. (We will cover the numbers game in Chapter 17.) These recommendations have changed several times throughout the decades, and there is no consensus between all medical, health, or nutrition professionals when it comes to these numbers. If it seems difficult to eat a high-quality diet that provides the RDA of calcium, for example, the problem may not be with the diet at all; perhaps the problem is with the RDA itself. In fact, an increasing number of health professionals are investigating this today. There is also a third area to consider when you hear someone pushing supplements or claiming our diets to be hopelessly inferior: their connection to any supplement sales. Many people who speak the loudest in favor of supplements, like multivitamins, are either directly or indirectly involved in their sales, so their stance on the topic should come as no surprise.

Of course, there is no question that today's food is not as nutrient rich as it was in the days before commercial farming, but with increased organic choices and a movement to grow our own food, this need not be a limiting factor for all. However, even if someone does not have access to any organic food but eats a whole-food, plant-based diet, they will still support their body in a much more beneficial way than someone who eats an inferior diet but takes a multivitamin. Any natural, whole-food, plant-based diet is abundantly nutrient rich, even more so if the foods come from local, organic, or homegrown sources.

The issues with multivitamins run deep. Some studies do show that they benefit various aspects of health, but others indicate that they actually harm, and still others show no effect either way. Can some people benefit from taking them? Most likely, but it all depends on the quality of the product, as well as a slew of other variables. What we do know for sure is that we cannot fix world hunger or malnutrition with multivitamins. Our bodies and health simply do not work this way. They require real, whole food.

If, for whatever reason, you do choose to use a multivitamin, be very vigilant about the brand and quality you buy. Most brands today are filled with numerous chemical and artificial ingredients. By way of example, here is a partial list of ingredients from one of the most popular multivitamin brands found in North America:

- Pregelatinized Corn Starch
- BHT
- Corn Starch
- Crospovidone
- FD&C Yellow No. 6 Aluminum Lake
- Gelatin
- Hydrogenated Palm Oil
- Hypromellose

- Modified Food Starch
- Polyethylene Glycol
- Polyvinyl Alcohol
- Silicon Dioxide
- Sodium Benzoate
- Stannous Chloride
- Sucrose
- Talc

You may recognize some of these ingredients, but I encourage you to look into some of those you are not familiar with. Does this list sound like something you should ingest for optimal health or to enhance your health? Hardly. Then why are we investing our money in products like this, because they are definitely not benefitting our health?

In the U.S., the FDA considers multivitamins a dietary supplement. This grants them exemption from the rigorous testing procedures required for pharmaceutical drugs; not that pharmaceutical drugs necessarily undergo credible testing but still. Any way we look at it, multivitamins have become a massive business. Synthetic multivitamin production began back in the 1940s and has only continued growing in popularity since. The original purpose of non-food vitamins and minerals was to treat deficiencies due to the lack of availability of certain foods. Today, the use of multivitamins tries to fix inferior diets that are based on processed food and has become quite indiscriminate, to say the least.

The problems associated with taking multivitamins become even more clear when we begin to understand the biochemistry of vitamins and minerals themselves. These compounds are very specific in how they work. Many of them either need each other to function properly or interfere with each other's function. This seems to be most obvious in synthetic and isolated forms of the compounds, not as they are naturally found in nature: as wholesome packets within our food. If calcium and iron, for example, inhibit one another, what can be gained by taking a product that includes them both? This is just one example of many that illustrates the intricate nature of these biochemical compounds.

Another concern is that many multivitamin products provide us with a quantity of these compounds far to high for a single taking. While our bodies may need some specific amount in a day, they do not need it all at once. The result is that many vitamins and minerals are excreted through the urine, and they can also add an unnecessary workload to our liver and kidneys. Additionally, regular reliance on multivitamins may wreak havoc when it comes to your body's ability to regulate and balance itself. It knows best what it needs and when, and adjusts accordingly in its extraction of it from the food we eat.

Taking one specific vitamin or mineral on its own is not always the way to go either. An overconsumption of any of these substances may block or inhibit the function of numerous others. The best way to take supplementary vitamins and minerals is under appropriate supervision of a natural health provider, like a naturopath or orthomolecular doctor. This way, your needs will be specifically tailored for a synergistic rather than antagonistic effect, ensuring the most benefit and the least harm. This can save your liver, your kidneys, and your wallet. Ultimately, a good healthcare physician will always try to point you in the direction of food before any pills, to resolve any health imbalances.

We are learning today that vitamins and minerals in our food do not act the same as their synthetic counterparts. When isolated from the whole food from which they were derived or synthesized, these synthetic compounds often have unpredictable effects. At best, they may offer some benefit or simply remain somewhat neutral. At worst, they can have negative effects on our health and wellbeing. Our system is equipped to handle these compounds most optimally when they come into our bodies in whole food form rather than in single or multiple, isolated, synthetic forms. Synthetic vitamins and minerals can contribute to various states of toxicity or irritating inner tissues, whereas vitamins and minerals from whole food do not pose these same risks. Researchers are finding that our bodies do not digest or absorb synthetic vitamins and minerals in the same way as those from whole food either. Vitamin and mineral biochemistry is very complex. We need to take into consideration the various forms of vitamins, as well as whether a mineral is coming in its organic or inorganic form, etc. (*Organic* is used here in a chemistry context, not a natural-farming context.)This is why we must be consciously discerning when it comes to any scientific conclusions drawn about these substances. Are sources talking about synthetic vitamins and minerals or whole-food vitamins and minerals? The answer is important, because the two are very different when it comes to how they will function within our bodies.

In his book, *Whole: Rethinking the Science of Nutrition*, Dr. T. Colin Campbell shares some of the research of one of his colleagues, Dr. Rui Hai Liu. Professor Liu chose to study the apple and its effects, given its popular association with good health. He began with an examination of its Vitamin C antioxidant activity. By focusing on this area, his research team made some startling discoveries, and these were published in the scientific journal, *Nature*.[3]

The research team found that 100 grams (about half an apple) had a Vitamin C-like antioxidant activity equivalent to 1,500mg of Vitamin C. When the apple was chemically analyzed, it was discovered that it only contained 5.7mg of actual Vitamin C. The practical implications of this are huge! First of all, it presents to us the power of whole, fresh, living plant food. The whole, fresh apple was 263 times more powerful in its Vitamin C-like activity than the isolated Vitamin C. This research shows that nearly all the antioxidant activity from apples comes from a variety of other compounds, which synthetic pills cannot replace or replicate with the perfection with which nature has created them. It also further illustrates the complex nature of vitamins when it comes to their characteristics and interactions. Modern science loves to find a beneficial ingredient in some plant food, then extract, isolate, and bottle it for our use. They may think they have done a good thing, but our bodies and nature simply do not work this way. There is a reason why whole, natural plant food looks and tastes the way it does, offering us unsurpassable benefits during its consumption.

Second, imagine if the apple was to be slapped with a nutrition facts label. (For your reference, store-bought bagged apples do contain them.) What would it say, in respect to how much Vitamin C it will provide per serving? Given that the current recommended Vitamin C range is 60 to 90mg per day, that would mean your apple serving would provide you with only 6 to 9.5 percent of your daily Vitamin C intake. Not too impressive, when in fact the apple easily surpassed the minimum requirement while providing you with many extra health benefits. This research also shows the powerful potential of natural antioxidants from fresh fruit versus isolated dietary supplements. To date, other research has shown that apples contain a wide variety of phytonutrients, many of which have been found to have strong antioxidant and anticancer properties and help reduce the risk of chronic disease. The take-home message is simple: Indeed, there is great truth in the age-old saying, "An apple a day keeps the doctor away." The best part is that it is not limited to apples; all whole, fresh plant foods hold similar potential and power for our health.

Vitamins and minerals *are* highly valuable and beneficial for optimal health but not necessarily when they are isolated and thrown together into a synthetic substance, along with other chemicals. Yes, we have made some wonderful progress in the field of health, thanks to vitamin and mineral supplements being able to correct various deficiencies. We even have a field called *orthomolecular* medicine, pertaining to the right molecule, which focuses on healing conditions using specific vitamins or minerals, in personalized and controlled dosages. This area was initiated by the work of Nobel Prize winner Linus Pauling during the latter part of the twentieth century. Since then, some natural health practitioners have been successfully using nutrient therapy to treat everything from cancer to depression. There is no doubt that this is all extremely valuable and should in no way be negated. We simply have to understand the parameters within which these substances work to make them most effective for our health, healing, and prevention.

Taking a multivitamin with a generic amount of vitamins and minerals from isolated, synthetic forms is far from conducive, as one size does not fit all. A thirty-five-year-old smoker who eats fast food is not going to require or benefit from the same amounts of vitamins and minerals as a thirty-five-year-old runner who eats whole food. We must be mindful of our personal needs rather than just blindly following the crowd. Look for all the nutrients you need in your food first and only follow up with a multivitamin if you find that the benefits will outweigh any disadvantages.

Practical Tips for Using Multivitamins

1. Synthetic multivitamins should never be taken on an empty stomach or simply with a glass of water. They should be taken with food for the most effective digestion and to prevent tissue irritation. (Some whole food-based multivitamins may be okay on an empty stomach. Read all package labels and instructions.)

2. Instead of a multivitamin, find out which vitamins or minerals your health would most benefit from or which you may be deficient in, and only take them under the guidance of your natural health provider.

3. Instead of a multivitamin, consider highly nutrient-dense food options that will provide a wide spectrum of vitamins and minerals in small amounts. Foods like chia seeds are a great example, as they are packed with vitamins, minerals, essential fatty acids, protein, fiber, and more.

4. Instead of a multivitamin, consider a high-quality, whole-food meal enhancement or replacement option when needed. Both Vega and Garden of Life provide whole-food, powdered shake products of outstanding quality and purity. While these can be very helpful during times of extreme stress or travel, remember that they are not a suitable replacement for an optimally healthy diet based on whole, real food.

5. If you choose to take a multivitamin, only invest your money and health in the highest quality possible. The product must offer vitamins and minerals taken from natural, whole-food sources rather than synthetic ones. The product should also be devoid of added colors, flavors, sugars, fillers, preservatives, or genetically modified ingredients. Garden of Life, MegaFood, and New Chapter are top choices within the very limited area of high-quality supplement considerations.

6. Always read all the ingredients, active and inactive, of your multivitamin to make sure it does not include any added colors, flavors, sugars (natural or artificial), fillers, preservatives, or genetically modified ingredients. Specific groups, such as those who have a gluten or lactose intolerance, as well as vegans or vegetarians, need to be extra mindful of the ingredients used and how the vitamins and minerals were sourced.

Fish Oils & Omega-3 Supplements

According to the "National Health Statistics Report" of 2008, fish oils and other omega-3 derivatives were the most commonly used non-vitamin/non-mineral dietary supplements amongst U.S. adults, with 37 percent of adults reporting their use in 2007. The 2013 *Council for Responsible Nutrition* consumer survey on dietary supplements found omega-3 and fish oils to be the third most commonly used supplement with about 19 percent of U.S. adults reporting their use. Although a significant drop appears within that six-year timeframe, the popularity of fish oil supplements continues to hold strong for the most part. However, is the popularity of these products justified when it comes to our health and resources? Let's explore.

As the increased prevalence of heart disease took front and center stage over the past several decades, omega-3 fatty acids appeared to be the magic bullet of protection and prevention. They have also been promoted to ease inflammation, improve mental health, decrease the risk of some cancers, and lengthen life. We have been told we are not getting enough omega-3 fatty acids, that we need more in our diets, and that they offer various health benefits. Many people jumped on the fish oil bandwagon, especially when reports of fish contamination began to be on the rise. It was claimed that fish oils were safe from heavy metal contamination.

Those were the general, mainstream messages that were shared, but the science of the matter proved to be much more complex. If you choose to look into this topic more thoroughly, you will find an abundance of studies that are completely contradictory when it comes to any benefits associated with omega-3 supplements, specifically fish oils. Some studies appear to show benefits for some areas of our health, while others show disadvantages for certain areas. Clearly, we cannot take supplements to help one thing if they are going to harm another. To do so would be counterintuitive. Still, despite the mixed messages, many people still religiously purchase and consume fish oil supplements.

A commonly held belief is that omega-3 supplementation can help protect against certain cancers. The research on this, however, has offered mixed results and has been inconclusive at best. Some studies report omega-3 fatty acids to be protective against some cancers, others report no association either way, and still others report a negative association. For example, a 2013 study by scientists at the Fred Hutchinson Cancer Research Center in Seattle linked eating a lot of oily fish or taking potent fish oil supplements to a 43 percent increased risk for prostate cancer overall and a 71 percent increased risk for aggressive prostate cancer.[4]

Even when it comes to cardiovascular health, the research is inconclusive and has many researchers looking in opposite directions. For example, a 2013 study published in the *New England Journal of Medicine* showed that omega-3 fatty acid supplements did nothing to reduce heart attacks, strokes, or deaths from heart disease in people with risk factors for heart disease.[5] The conclusion with this group of supplements seems to be the same as we saw in the multivitamin section: Isolated nutrients are incapable of replacing whole-food nutrients and act in imperfect, unpredictable ways that can create more harm than good.

When it comes to the quality of these supplements, reports have brought important concerns to light about the lack of quality control in this area. Due to the sensitive nature of these supplements, specific handling and processing must be applied. Some fish oil brands show distinct mercury contamination. Thus, we can no longer hold on to the belief that only whole fish are prone to chemical contamination; the supplements made from them can be as well. Another cause for concern is the lack of adequate freshness. A 2010 Norwegian government-sponsored study by Nofima, a food research institute, reported that upward of 95 percent of omega-3 supplements on the market don't meet industry standards for freshness and contain excessively oxidized oil.[6] Rancid oils are, in fact, inflammatory and damaging to our bodies and health, doing the very opposite of what these supplements are intended for. Therefore, great care must be taken in the selection process if one is going to choose to use these supplements. Like any other popular industry, this one is not exempt from poor-quality products and unsubstantiated hype infiltrating it.

Do we really need a fish oil supplement, especially if we choose not to eat fish? The answer is, by no means, a definitive yes. As with all areas of health and nutrition, we need to undertake a more in-depth analysis of all relevant areas. Understanding the overall quality of our diet and health, as well as the biochemistry of these essential fatty acids, is necessary before we can make the most informed decisions. Research what various sources have to say about this topic to gain the most objective view, and discuss as needed with your natural or integrative healthcare provider.

Omega-3 is a family of fats from the polyunsaturated group. Within this family are three most noteworthy essential fatty acids: alpha-linolenic acid (ALA), as well as eicosapentaenoic acid (EPA) and docosahexaenoic acid (DHA). These fatty acids play important roles in brain function, normal growth, development, and regulation of inflammation. Deficiencies have been linked to numerous health problems, but this does not necessarily mean that ingesting these fatty acids in an isolated form and high doses is good for our health or disease prevention, as we have just finished discussing.

ALA is considered an essential fatty acid because our bodies do not manufacture it; therefore, we must obtain it from our diet. Flax, chia, and hemp seeds and their oil; walnuts; dark green, leafy vegetables; squash; beans; and soy are excellent sources of ALA. EPA and DHA are not quite essential but usually treated as such, and thus, considered very important. If our diet has sufficient ALA, our bodies are designed to convert ALA into EPA, then EPA into DHA. In most healthy individuals, with high-quality natural, whole-food, plant-based diets, this conversion process should work as intended. If it is compromised in any way, such as lack of sufficient ALA and/or too much omega-6 fatty acids in the diet from refined oils, processed, or animal foods, the conversion may be blocked or inadequate, at which time EPA and DHA must come from external sources.

Many experts today insist that eating ALA-rich foods alone is not enough and that fish or fish oils must be consumed. They claim the conversion rate in the body is not efficient or high enough and, therefore, is not adequate to give us enough EPA or DHA to maintain good health and protect us from future health issues. However, there is another big piece to this puzzle. The quickest way to compromise the ALA-to-EPA-to-DHA conversion pathway is to eat a diet high in omega-6, specifically linoleic acid (LA). Omega-3 och Hälsa, an independent-testing Swedish group, explains that it is unknown how efficient this transformation is, as studies have shown different results. A limiting factor is that the same enzymes are used to transform both LA (omega-6) and ALA (omega-3) fatty acids, but this cannot be done simultaneously.[7] This creates competition for these enzymes, and if the diet is overly high in omega-6, it appears that this greatly inhibits proper omega-3 fatty acid conversion. What we do know for sure is that the standard American diet (SAD) is very high in omega-6 fatty acids. If you have been eating a diet based on refined oils, processed foods, and animal products, you can be sure you've been getting an abundance of omega-6 fatty acids and lacking omega-3 fatty acids. It is estimated most people today eat a ratio of anywhere from ten to fifty omega-6 fatty acids to one omega-3 fatty acids. Anthropological, epidemiological, and studies at the molecular level indicate that human beings evolved on a diet with a ratio of omega-6 to omega-3 of approximately one to one.[8] Ideally, we should not go beyond a ratio of three to one omega-6 to omega-3 fatty acids. Diets high in omega-6 are inflammatory in nature, leading to all sorts of health problems and degenerative conditions.

Our approach to solve these health problems in the population has been predictable. Instead of being given a solution at the root level via our diet, such as being taught about the consequences of high-omega-6 diets and taught practical ways of reducing them, we are told to buy a new product to remedy the problem. Through the use of isolated nutrients, we are supposed to help our bodies balance this ratio and benefit our health. Of course, we could just go straight to whole-food fish sources, but given today's contamination problems and severely imbalanced diets, high fish consumption can easily lead to a host of other problems. Hence, we struggle to get enough omega-3 fatty acids to offset the high omega-6 effects, when the easier solution would be to reduce the omega-6 amounts in our diet. There is no doubt that the key to optimizing our health in this area lies in optimizing the omega-6:omega-3 ratio. When we make the conscious choice to eat whole, natural, plant-based food, as shared in this book, we set our bodies up for good health. If we choose to consume a diet based on fried and greasy foods, refined oils and lard, and processed and animal foods, we set our bodies up for a state of disease.

At the end of the day, whether you really need an omega-3 supplement, regardless of what form it takes—fish oil or microalgae (root source of DHA) or other EPA or DHA supplement—should be a well-thought-out and researched decision. Consult with your natural healthcare provider, and work primarily with your diet to provide you with the most appropriate healing and prevention. It is easy to consume a diet rich in omega-3 fatty acids and adequate in omega-6 fatty acids by following the guidelines shared in this book. The whole premise of this dietary lifestyle is that it is naturally anti-cancerous, anti-inflammatory, and supportive for the cardiovascular system. We can get a lot more value and protection from the type of foods we eat than from any pill we take.

Practical Tips for Using Fish Oils

1. If you choose to use a fish oil supplement, research the best brands that have the highest reputation for quality and purity. Fish oils often go rancid. The color, texture, and odor must all be examined. Transparent yellow, firm capsules that have a mild fish smell, if any, can be presumed to be non-rancid oils. The worst case scenario with these products is not that they do not work, but that they harm your health. You are investing both your health and money, so making the best choice is vital.

2. If you choose to use a fish oil supplement, consider krill rather than fish oil. These appear to have more benefits and less contamination issues.

3. If you want to bypass the whole fish oil dilemma, consider microalgae supplements, which have less problems than their animal counterparts when it comes to any kind of contamination issues. These are especially useful if pregnant or nursing, as they will help you avoid mercury exposure. They are also the top choice for vegans/vegetarians.

4. Avoid fish oil supplements that contain any colors, flavors, GMO ingredients, preservatives, or other additives, which are not optimal for your health.

Vitamin D

Up to the twenty-first century, Vitamin D was mainly associated with its role in the healing and prevention of Rickets, a condition associated with bone deformity due to inadequate mineralization in growing bones. Since the turn of this century, Vitamin D has been steadily gaining attention, due to its role in all areas of our health, including healing and prevention of cancer. The 2013 Council for Responsible Nutrition consumer survey on dietary supplements found Vitamin D to be the second most commonly used supplement, with about 20 percent of U.S. adults reporting its use. In fact, today's natural health experts recommend that the majority of the population living in northern areas should be supplementing regularly with Vitamin D.

When it comes to quantity, it wasn't that long ago that we were told we only need about 400 IU daily. Today, that number has risen drastically. Depending on which expert you consult, recommendations range anywhere from 1,000 to 10,000 IU per day. The reason for this is twofold. First, ongoing research about the role of Vitamin D, with respect to various degenerative diseases, continues to link it to being highly healing and protective. It has been correlated with having a positive effect on the healing and prevention of cancer, osteoporosis, heart disease, multiple sclerosis, depression, as well as being highly supportive for our immune system and overall health. The second reason deals with the reported epidemic of Vitamin D deficiency in the global population. Various estimates share that anywhere from 40 to 90 percent of the population is

Vitamin D deficient. This varies so widely, based on what markers and population demographics are used. Either way, there is a clear problem in the population, with too many people being low in this critical compound.

You may be wondering how such a drastic deficiency came about, especially today, given our modern and technologically advanced way of life. The possible causes span many areas with those modern technological advances actually being part of the problem. This is related to our relationship with the sun or lack thereof. For the past few decades, we have been told to cover up and stay out of the sun. This is ironic, considering that the sun is our best, most trusted, most natural source of the hormone-like Vitamin D, and conclusive results about the sun's role in the proliferation of skin cancer have not been made. As always, there is so much more to this story. We will not get into the issues of sunscreen safety or the misleading logic about its use here, nor will we discuss the numerous variables that affect different types of skin cancer and its occurrence. However, it can be said that this phenomenon, along with Vitamin D not being found in many foods and our highly indoor-bound lifestyles, are very likely why we are having the magnitude of deficiencies we are now facing. Our connection with nature, the sun, and all the natural elements has been greatly marginalized, and our health is clearly showing us the consequences.

It is also necessary to consider geographic location, as there is a distinct difference in the Vitamin D-producing ray amount and intensity, depending on where we live. It varies mainly by season and latitude. In our modern world, we have pushed the limits of nature and today inhabit many areas where it is naturally more challenging to survive, never mind thrive. Thanks to our advanced heating and cooling systems, as well as our transportation and technology, we have been able to expand our habitats over many areas of our planet. There need not be anything inherently wrong with this approach, as long as we realize its limits and address those accordingly. This is where a supplemental Vitamin D is almost always a wise choice for those living in the northern climates.

Despite our apparent need to rely on this isolated nutrient, we should still take steps in our daily lives to ensure that its most natural form is our first choice. Start by re-establishing a smart, respectful relationship with the sun. The sun has been the source of life and vitality from the beginning of time, and it is foolish for us to think we can today thrive without it. We must make regular sun exposure, especially during peak Vitamin D production times, a priority in our life, just like we will our food. Second, it may be valuable to have a blood test to determine your Vitamin D levels. This can be done annually if you have deficiency concerns or every few years if your health, diet, and lifestyle is top notch. Based on your results, you will know how much of a Vitamin D supplement will be the best option for you. Consult with a trusted natural healthcare provider to optimize your Vitamin D levels.

Practical Tips for Using Vitamin D

1. Vitamin D is most commonly sold in the D2 (fungus-derived) and D3 (animal-derived) form. Vegans and vegetarians will want to be especially mindful of this. (There is a brand called Vitashine that sources D3 from lichen for vegans and vegetarians.)

2. Aside from the origin, there is still some debate in regard to the efficiency and bioavailability of D2 compared to D3. Most supplements on the market are in the most commonly recommended form, D3, but it is not uncommon to find foods or supplement formulas fortified with D2.

3. The hormone-like D is a fat-soluble vitamin, so it should be taken with meals that have a healthy fat content, not simply with water on an empty stomach.

4. Avoid Vitamin D supplements that contain any colors, flavors, GMO ingredients, preservatives, or other additives, which are not optimal for your health.

5. As covered in Chapter 14, mushrooms are increasingly linked with being a reliable source of Vitamin D. Many mushrooms naturally contain this vitamin, and studies show that mushrooms exposed to ultraviolet light are able to synthesize this vitamin very efficiently. There have also been reports about some Vitamin D content in hemp seeds. Keep an eye out for new research in this area. I have no doubt that this will provide more options for us to consume Vitamin D in more optimal ways, aside from the most natural way from the sun.

Calcium

Calcium has also become one of the fastest-growing, most popular supplements used. The 2013 Council for Responsible Nutrition consumer survey on dietary supplements found calcium to be the fourth most commonly used supplement, with about 18 percent of U.S. adults reporting its use. As we covered in the acid-alkaline section of Chapter 4, the theories we hold about dairy, calcium, and bone health are often incomplete.

It is outside the scope of this book to cover the complex physical and biochemical aspects of how diet, exercise, and calcium consumption interact for best bone density and strength. There are many variables to consider, such as age, sex, diet, movement, race, etc. Bone-density testing tools and protocols are also debated and controversial with respect to their value, accuracy, and effectiveness. What we can say with certainty is that we should always start with the root approach rather than the surface, just putting on a Band-aid. This means focusing on diet and exercise as the primary ways to build and maintain proper bone strength and density. Physical movement, anything from walking to various weight-bearing exercises, yoga included, is one of the best ways to increase and maintain our bone strength and density throughout our lifetime. With our diet, the first step is to achieve an acid-alkaline balance so that our bodies do not need to leach calcium and other bone-building minerals from our bones to offset an acidic lifestyle (refer to Chapter 4). The healing and prevention lifestyle outlined in this book is fully supportive for strong and healthy bones; greens are amongst the top sources of bioavailable calcium and nearly all whole, plant foods are a source of calcium. It is much more important to focus on overall dietary excellence than try to aim for the artificial numbers that try to declare how much calcium we need each day. As previously mentioned, these numbers continue to be questioned by numerous health experts, as do the isolated forms and amounts of calcium supplements recommended. If this topic is of pertinent interest to you, I recommend the work of Dr. Pamela Popper, the Executive Director of The Wellness Forum, who is an internationally-recognized expert on bone health and dietary excellence.

The bottom line is that bone health goes far beyond calcium intake. Vitamins D, C, K, magnesium, and phosphorus are just some of the major key players when it comes to optimal bone health. Like with the essential fatty acid ratio we just talked about, it is necessary to examine our calcium:magnesium and calcium:Vitamin D ratios when addressing proper bone health. It takes a whole team, not a single player, to achieve a successful outcome. Calcium supplements have also been linked to various health problems, including kidney stones, arthritis, and hardening of the arteries, just to name a few. Nutrition and natural health experts like David Wolfe regularly speak out about these dangers. Studies that support calcium supplements don't always measure the right values either. It is not about how much calcium gets into the bloodstream; we should be far more interested in how much of it actually makes it into the bone.

If you choose to take a calcium supplement, quality and purity are equally important considerations. The most common form, calcium carbonate, is also the most problematic. So, whether a calcium supplement is right for you, which type and how much should be discussed with a trusted natural healthcare provider.

Practical Tips for Using Calcium

1. If you must take a calcium supplement, choose calcium citrate or chelate over calcium carbonate. Calcium carbonate is harder to digest and has been linked to contamination and health problems.

2. Take small quantities more frequently rather than one major dose daily. Our bodies don't absorb large doses of calcium as efficiently as small ones. Thus, 250 mg tablets spread out over the day are better than a single 500 mg or 1000 mg tablet.

3. Avoid calcium supplements that come in forms like chewy squares or flavored, candy-like options. These contain various unnecessary and harmful ingredients, like refined sugars, artificial sugars, flavors, fillers, colors, and preservatives.

4. Work on optimizing your diet first, and incorporate healthy movement before relying on calcium supplements. It is much more beneficial to remove foods and drinks from your diet that tax your body's calcium supplies, than to add in synthetic and/or isolated calcium.

Vitamin B12

For those who choose to take their diet to the next level and go 100 percent plant-based, whether temporarily or permanently, it is a good idea to consider a Vitamin B12 supplement. In fact, it appears that many people in the population today, regardless of how much meat, eggs, or dairy they consume, would benefit from vitamin B12. Vitamin B12 originates from bacteria in soil or water. When animals feed, their food naturally contains this bacteria. This has contributed to how humans have obtained our Vitamin B12 through the ages. Due to modern farming practices and strict sanitary habits, we no longer get this bacteria from nature like the animals do—at least not in amounts that seem to be adequate, unless one is consuming a very natural, homegrown, organic diet and/or drinking from natural springs. In fact, as we age, regardless of our dietary choices, we seem to have more trouble absorbing this vitamin. Various biochemical factors play a role in this occurrence and for some people, the problems start even as early as their teens. If you have any concerns, get annual blood work done to monitor your levels of Vitamin B12.

B12 levels normally take years to deteriorate since the body is very efficient at recycling it. Nevertheless, it is wise to stay attentive to your needs as vitamin B12 deficiency has serious consequences for many areas of our health, especially our nervous system. Unchecked, long-term deficiencies can result in conditions like pernicious anemia or even permanent health damage. Based on your blood results and dietary choices, if there is a need for a B12 supplement, it is important to know which one to choose and the correct dosage. Consult a trusted natural healthcare provider to optimize the use of this vitamin as needed.

Practical Tips for Using Vitamin B12

1. Vitamin B12 comes in several forms. While cyanocobalamin is the most common, methylcobalamin appears to be most beneficial, which is the active form of the vitamin.

2. It is best to take this vitamin sublingually (under the tongue), as is the case with methylcobalamin, rather than orally, by swallowing. This allows it to

be absorbed in a more efficient manner; it bypasses the digestive tract, where it can commonly be destroyed.

3. Remember that some foods, like certain varieties of nutritional yeast and mushrooms, may be reliable sources of Vitamin B12. Explore possible options.

Herbal Supplements

Plants have been used as medicine since the beginning of human time as we know it. For thousands of years, they have served as natural healing remedies for all sorts of ills and ailments, big and small. Many indigenous cultures to this day depend on them and know how to appropriately harness the rich medicinal compounds found in plants. For the rest of the world, however, when the modern-day pharmaceutical industry took over, natural herbal remedies pretty much went out the window. After all, if they cannot be patented, they are not very good for business.

Since the start of the twenty-first century, we have seen a shift back to natural herbal remedies, especially as the supplement industry has grown. This has also seen more people coming back to benefit from the many medicinal and healing characteristics of plants. Today, we have many herbal supplements to choose from, but as we now know, this can be both a positive and negative aspect. It is wonderful that we have fairly easy access to numerous herbal supplements that can be used for both healing and prevention. However, it can be harmful or wasteful if we underestimate the power of plant medicines and use them indiscriminately or if we self-medicate without appropriate information or buy herbal products of an inferior quality. When needing or wanting to use an herbal supplement, it is best to research and/or consult a trusted natural health provider who is an expert in this field, and always choose the highest, pure-quality versions. Remember that herbal remedies come from plants that may have been grown with pesticides or synthetic fertilizers; this will impact the quality of the product and its effect on you. Therefore, choose pure, organic options.

Other Supplements

There are numerous other supplements out there that do not fit neatly into any of the categories we have talked about thus far. The supplements industry is a large and powerful one, and many want to push their products into the market or ride the wave of the latest nutritional hype or diet fad. While I do not discount that there are some supplements that can aid our health and be used for healing many conditions as an alternative to pharmaceutical drugs, I must also pass along a word of caution. Many supplements are marketed as being the answer to your problems. If this were so, our health and weight would not be in such a grim condition. Therefore, be wary of miracle claims. It may be tempting or seem easy, but there truly is no quick fix if we are serious about optimal health. Your diet should always—and I stress again, *always*—come first in preventing and healing any conditions. Don't fall for the false sense of security you think you will find in a bottle, something that you think will let you off the hook from pursuing dietary excellence. Too many products on the market today are inadequately tested, if at all, others include synthetic or unfavorable ingredients, and far too many are, plainly put, a waste of your money. Whatever supplement you may be interested in, always opt for its original source first. For example, instead of maca capsules, choose real, ground maca root; instead of resveratrol capsules, choose organic, red grapes and other whole foods rich in this compound.

There are two other supplements I wish to share with you that are actually considered food at their basic level: spirulina and chlorella. These microscopic plants, microalgae, grow in fresh water. They can be considered nutritional supplements or superfoods or functional foods. Spirulina and chlorella have a lot in common. Both are nutritionally dense and contain vitamins, minerals, essential fatty acids, protein, nucleic acids (RNA and DNA), chlorophyll, and a vast spectrum of phytonutrients. This makes them a much more natural option to consider for getting vitamins and minerals over commercial multivitamins. They contain a high-quality protein that is more dense and digestible than any animal-derived protein. Both are also highly detoxifying and have a long list of health benefits that include: supporting our healing, cleansing, healthy aging, immune system, and significantly lowering cancer risk. They are anti-inflammatory and activate cell renewal. Although they are similar and can both be enjoyed, small differences exist that may make you choose one over the other, based on your needs. I encourage you to look into both of these foods to see if or how they can benefit you on your journey of healing and prevention. If you ever choose to use either one, source them in their pure, powdered forms rather than any pill form. These can be easily added to smoothies or even some of your healthy snacks as presented in Chapter 15.

In the end, to prevent or heal disease, we need to look at our food. Our best external health insurance policy is not pills. Rather, it is the food we eat daily.

CHAPTER 17
The Numbers Game

The science of nutrition has been on an ever-accelerating and expanding journey since about the 1800s and was highly influenced by Newtonian or reductionist science. It is important to highlight this latter point, as it will help us understand our fixation on details, numbers, and isolated parts where our food and nutrition is concerned.

As far as we know, humans and other animals have engaged in nourishment through the consumption of various foods since the beginning. Food was seen as a form of survival, growth, energy, and strength, as well as an element of commerce and celebration. However, something drastically began to change about 200 years ago. As our scientific and technological advancements began to flourish, we began to study our food and dissect it into ever smaller parts. We were thrilled with the depth and understanding this provided. All of a sudden, we could actually see some of the connections between what we ate and the diseases that plagued us, especially the post-Industrial Revolution societies. This newfound knowledge brought about a sense of empowerment and control.

We began in the early 1800s by learning the simple, chemical composition of food. We discovered that foods are composed primarily of four elements: carbon, nitrogen, hydrogen, and oxygen. By the end of the 1800s, we had a basic understanding of the macronutrients: carbohydrates, fats, and proteins. Then, around the early to mid-1900s, we grasped an understanding of micronutrients, the vitamins and minerals. The early period of the twentieth century came to be known as the Golden Age of Nutrition, giving way to numerous important discoveries and scientific advancements within the field of nutritional science. These would shape and influence our relationship with food for decades to come, for better and worse. Finally, around the 1980s, the science of nutrition began to identify yet another important food component, one found specifically in plant food. This nutrient group came to be known as the phytochemicals (or phytonutrients), from Greek *phuton* meaning "a plant." We learned (and are still learning) that there are thousands of these bioactive compounds, and they are proving to be highly beneficial for our health. This area of nutritional science is still in its early stages of understanding, and we are still learning how powerful whole plant foods are for our healing and prevention, due to the presence of these phytonutrients.

Going back to the late 1800s, it was around this time that Wilbur Atwate, the Father of Nutritional Science, along with his team of scientists, established estimates for the metabolizable energy of carbohydrates, protein, and fat as four, four, and nine kcal/g respectively. They carried out tests to measure the energy provided by food and created a system to measure this energy in units, what we know as food calories. Thus began the era of calories and macronutrient compositions.

Given all these advancements in the field of nutrition and the excitement each discovery brought forth, we went deeper and deeper into quantifying isolated nutrients and trying to understand their effects on our health. Once basic connections were made between nutrients and the presence of health or disease, our focus shifted to numbers. Although the USDA (established in 1862) had come up with some basic nutrient quantity requirements, it was during World War II that the RDA was developed by the United States National Academy of Sciences. What many may find surprising is that its intention was to investigate issues of nutrition that might "affect national defense," specifically for the armed forces, civilians, and overseas population who needed food relief. It was for this primary reason that the committee began to deliberate on a set of recommendations of a standard daily allowance for each type of nutrient. The allowances were meant to provide superior nutrition for civilians and military personnel, so they included a "margin of safety." The Food and Nutrition Board has subsequently revised the RDAs every five to ten years. In 1997, the dietary reference intake (DRI) was introduced in order to broaden the existing RDA guidelines.

Calories

When it comes to the numbers game, calories are among the most popular of digits that are examined. For the past few decades, especially as excess weight became such a prevalent phenomenon in our society, the focus turned to managing calories. Above, we learned that each macronutrient is worth a certain amount of calories. Based on simple science, it was believed that energy input versus energy output was the main component in determining whether someone would lose, gain, or simply maintain their weight. We passionately embraced the idea of counting calories and paid a lot of attention to them, in the hopes that they would be the solution to our weight problems.

As it turns out, however, all calories are far from equal. Today, this is a well-known fact, but it has not yet circulated deeply into the mainstream. The truth is that 100 calories of a refined cookie are in no way equivalent to 100 calories of fresh fruit. Sure, both will provide you with a similar amount of energy, but—and this is a big one—how your body will digest and utilize that food, as well as the effect of this food on your body, will be very different. The refined cookie provides very little value, if any at all, but it does harbor a lot of problematic characteristics. The fresh fruit provides lots of value and, generally speaking, no drawbacks. How each of those foods will impact your organs, your immune system, your acid-alkaline balance, and so on will all play a role in whether you gain, lose, or maintain your weight, not to mention your health. Our bodies are not just looking for energy in the form of calories; they are also looking for nutrients. When our foods do not provide us with these crucial nutrients and additionally introduce stress and problems, imbalances occur in our weight and health.

There is no doubt that many people, if not most, eat too much today, and they often eat too much of the wrong stuff—the pseudo foods, as I like to call them. Yes, too many calories from almost any food can result in excess weight; however, all the calorie-counting in the world is not going to create optimal weight or health for us. Your body simply does not function in such a simplistic way. Thus, it is futile to get wrapped up in the calorie-counting numbers game. As we talked about in Chapters 2 and 3, we should focus on real, whole foods—specifically plant foods—because they naturally come with a high nutrient density, providing lots of nutrients in exchange for few calories. This allows us to enjoy our food without having to worry about counting calories, and it is part of nature's innate intelligence, its very design. On the other hand, processed and refined foods come with very few nutrients and a heaping helping of calories. This is why we have to be smart about our food selection and focus on nutrient density as the guiding factor for our dietary choices to get the most for our health, our weight, and our dollars.

Carbohydrates

Carbohydrates are the main fuel source for our bodies, especially our brain. This is basic biology as we have come to know it. Just like a machine will run optimally with the right kind of fuel, your body will run properly with glucose. Can your body run on other fuels, such as fats or proteins? Yes, but there is always a cost to consider, such as the consequences of biochemical conversion. Imagine trying to run your car on a different fuel, and you will quickly understand that the consequences may be anywhere from minimally to seriously problematic. Over the last few decades, carbohydrates have been vilified and their importance downgraded, depending on the particulars of various fad diets. Just like other areas of nutrition, misinformation and lack of proper understanding has led to problems and confusion for many people when it comes to carbs.

Carbohydrates, as a nutrient group, are neither bad nor good. It all depends on what carbohydrates we are talking about and from what sources they come. This group includes complex carbohydrates (starches), simple carbohydrates (sugars), and fiber. Whole, natural food sources will provide the different types of these carbohydrates in their healthy forms, those our bodies are most optimized to utilize. Fruits, vegetables, grains, and beans are all rich sources of healthy carbohydrates when it comes to their starch, sugar, and fiber compositions. Hopefully, this will trigger you to see the inherent problem with low- and zero-carb diets. Such diets not only limit or eliminate core nutrients that your body needs, but also the beneficial foods that are their main source. All whole, natural plant and fungi foods are, to some degree, a source of carbohydrates. On the contrary, most animal foods have zero to very few, and all are completely devoid of fiber.

The biggest problem with carbohydrates is in their refinement. As we covered in Parts 1 and 2 of this book, refined versions of our whole, natural foods should be avoided for optimal health, weight, healing, and prevention. This includes refined carbohydrates, fats, and proteins. Refined foods are often rich sources of refined carbohydrates, especially refined sugars. Additionally, flour-based products, even when whole, tend to act like sugars in our bodies. This leads to all sorts of imbalances, like unhealthy blood glucose levels and strain on various organs and systems. Diets that frequently cause our blood sugar to spike, remain high, or imbalanced are extremely problematic for our weight and destructive to our health.

In terms of numbers given for this nutrient, depending on the source you consult, recommendations suggest that anywhere from 40 to 80 percent of our calories should come from carbohydrates. The FAO/WHO states that an optimum diet should consist of at least 55 percent of total energy from a variety of carbohydrate sources. According to the 2002 "Dietary Reference Intakes for Energy, Carbohydrate, Fiber, Fat, Fatty Acids, Cholesterol, Protein, and Amino Acids," adults should get 45 to 65 percent of their calories from carbohydrates. Many holistic and natural health guidelines advise a range of 60 to 80 percent. At first glance, some consider these numbers high, especially at the 80 percent mark, but when we remind ourselves that most of this should come from wholesome vegetables, there really is nothing too high about it. Vegetables are our primary sources of food for healing, prevention, and optimal weight maintenance, so they should be the primary focus of our meals. Any of the carb guidelines above, regardless of how low or high, can become a huge problem if the bulk of those carbohydrates come from refined sources, such as breads, boxed cereals, pastas, pizzas, waffles, crackers, chips, cookies, etc.

In terms of amounts in grams, the currently recommended carbohydrate numbers by the major health organizations (USDA and Health Canada) are set at 100g/day as the estimated average requirement (EAR) and 130g/day (RDA/AI). This has been determined to be the minimum required amount to provide the brain with an adequate supply of glucose. In practical terms, these values are low, as exemplified by the AMDR (acceptable macronutrient distribution range) or simple calculations. We cannot forget that they are based on minimum requirements. For most adults, normal carbohydrate intake is recommended to be in the 250 to 350g range. To compare these amounts, typical zero- or low-carb diets restrict participants to only 20g of carbohydrates per day!

In the end, as is the case with calories, the amount of carbohydrates you consume per day will not be the ultimate answer to optimal health and weight, and it would be a tedious waste of your time to try to count them. The essential task is simply to consume the right source of carbohydrates—real, whole plant foods—and to guide yourself naturally with those food choices each day.

Fats

Like carbohydrates, fats have gone through their own notorious journey. According to the American Heart Association, the U.S. obesity epidemic began in approximately 1980 and accelerated from 1990 to 2005. From the mid- to late 1900s, we also put a lot of focus on research about heart disease. Even though deaths from heart disease have been decreasing since the 1970s, cardiovascular disease, strokes, hypertension, and high cholesterol continue to be a major burden for our society. Thus, the focus turned to fat. It appeared logical that consuming too much fat would make us fat, clog our arteries, and contribute to heart disease. This message quickly rippled through all major health and nutrition organizations. In the late 1970s, the U.S. government started telling all Americans to eat less fat, and in the mid-1980s, the production of low-fat products began. What most overlooked at the time, and still do, to a degree, is that the calories in these foods generally remained the same. What changed was the fat composition of the refined foods (yogurts, sauces, spreads, dressings, dips, etc.), which was replaced with refined carbohydrates. Today, the consensus is pretty clear: low-fat does not equate to weight loss or healthy weight maintenance, nor do low-fat options offer necessary protection against heart disease. There is much more to this story.

The second part of the fat numbers game that needs to be considered is that, just like with carbs, we cannot vilify this nutrient group or simplistically label it as good or bad. Again, it all depends on what kind of fat we are talking about and from what food sources it comes. There are many different fatty acids with varying compositions and ratios within any given food, and each has unique effects on our health and weight. There are monounsaturated, polyunsaturated, and saturated sub-groups, yet even within those groups, vast differences dictate their effects on our health and weight. None of them can be collectively deemed good or bad. Related to fats, there is also the substance known as cholesterol. It, too, is neither good or bad, though most certainly a subject of numerous controversies itself. Our bodies naturally produce this substance in its various forms within healthy or unhealthy ranges depending on our diet and lifestyle (presence of exercise, stress, alcohol, cigarettes, etc.). Animal foods are the predominant source of exogenous cholesterol and it, along with unsaturated, saturated, and trans fats, influences our cholesterol levels.

When it comes to percentages, common guidelines recommend that anywhere from 10 to 30 percent of our calories come from fats. However, don't be surprised to find claims that recommend upward of 60 percent. Due to the fact that fat contains more than double the energy or calories per gram, a dietary difference in composition of our diet between just 10 and 20 percent can make a big difference. Not only do health and nutrition experts have trouble agreeing on what percentage of fat is best, but they are also not in consensus about what actually constitutes a low-fat diet. Some feel it would fall in the 10 percent range, while others claim that 30 percent is low fat. Another dilemma with these numbers is that they almost never specify what kind of fat or from what sources they are referring to. As I teach, we must first understand that there are four classifications of fat-focused diets:

1. **Natural Low-Fat** (ex: a whole-food, plant-based diet)

2. **Artificial Low-Fat** (ex: a refined-food diet based on low-fat products)

3. **Natural High-Fat** (ex: an Inuit or Weston Price diet)

4. **Artificial High-Fat** (ex: a refined-, fast food-, and/or animal-based diet)

As you can hopefully deduce based on reading this far, Options 2 and 4 will not generate optimal health or weight or healing and prevention. Option 3 may be healthful, but this depends on several variables, one of the main ones being the environment in which we live. The closer we live to the Equator or the warmer the area in which we live, the more we are guided to and benefit from a naturally low-fat diet. The further north we live or the colder the climate, the more we benefit from a naturally higher fat diet. For most of us in the modern world, this means eating a diet lower in fat throughout the spring and summer months and one higher in fat throughout the fall and winter months. No numbers or special prescriptions are necessary; if and when we mindfully connect with our body's needs, we will naturally be guided to the right food choices. Either way, whole, natural plant foods can perfectly satisfy both of these needs year round. We have to take into account as well that our lifestyles today are quite far removed from that of our ancestors. We spend the majority of our days indoors, lead sedentary lifestyles, and have pretty much any food available to us year round, with minimal effort. Therefore, as previously discussed, we cannot simply apply the dietary patterns of our ancestors or those living in indigenous communities without some serious discernment. As times change, as our bodies and lifestyles evolve; so, too, must our diets.

In terms of fat amounts in grams, the common, general recommendations advise us to get anywhere from 40 to 105g of fat per day. Sources recommend that saturated fat comprise less than 20g, about 7 percent of total calories per day. The World Health Organization and others, like the American Heart Association, recommend that the total amount of trans fats consumed be less than 1 percent of total calories per day, which will typically work out to less than 2g. Common guidelines given for cholesterol are for us to have less than 300mg per day.

As you might imagine, not all experts agree with these numbers, nor are they universally accepted, so don't put too much emphasis on them. It all goes back to the source of these fats. What foods do they come from? First, we need to consider animal versus plant fat sources, as this alone can clear up so much of the controversy surrounding fat values. Second, we need to consider the form these foods come in; if we are consuming mostly fried or refined fat foods, even hovering around the low end of the fat guidelines is not a smart choice for our health or weight. Third, we need to consider the quality of these foods; a lot of the animal foods that may have been healthful at one time now have unhealthy fat profiles due to the unnatural food and living conditions that the animals themselves are subjected to. Fourth, the overall quality of our diet and lifestyle influences how the type and quantity of fat we eat is processed by our body.

The full story of nutrition is vast, and many of the discrepancies go back to one of the first points I shared in this chapter: our reductionist approach to science and nutrition. We must swing the pendulum back into a more balanced space, where we consider the whole, big picture when it comes to our food. Whether it is carbs or fats, we cannot afford to get lost in isolated nutrients and the numbers game.

Proteins

"We never talk about protein anymore, because it's absolutely not an issue, even among children. If anything, we talk about the dangers of high-protein diets. Getting enough is simply a matter of getting enough calories."

— Marion Nestle, PhD, Chair of the Department of Nutrition
at New York University

Out of the three macronutrients, protein is the only one that has seemingly escaped negative controversy during the last 100 years. Like the Greek origin of its name, meaning "of prime importance," it has enjoyed an elevated status and has been portrayed as a nutrient that can do no possible harm. Whenever a new fad diet surfaces, it is generally focused on reducing fats and/or the carbohydrates; if protein is mentioned, it is to emphasize that we get more, not less, protein. Today, the tables are finally turning, as this is yet another misleading area of the numbers game on which we got hooked. Nearly all of us, at one time or another, have bought into the claims that high protein or more protein is good for us and that this nutrient is somehow limited in the food supply. Neither of these two beliefs are accurate. Before we look at the protein numbers, let's take a quick look back in history to see where, why, and how protein achieved such nutritional superiority.

During the 1900s, much research was done to gain an understanding of things like amino acids, nitrogen balance, and, ultimately, protein quality and quantity. The first problem here is that a lot of the research was carried out on animals, with animal foods. Both of these factors, in the midst of a reductionist mindset, created various faulty conclusions that have become deeply embedded in our society to this day. As we continued to study nutrition, more fuel was added to this fire when the attention turned to poverty-stricken, developing areas in the world, with a special emphasis on children. At first, it was believed that their extremely poor health was simply due to a protein deficiency. By the 1960s the

211

Food and Agriculture Organization (FAO) had declared protein research as its main goal. Nevertheless, it quite quickly became clear that protein was just one piece of the puzzle. Whether dealing with PEM (protein-energy malnutrition) or Kwashiorkor (a type of PEM focused predominantly on protein malnutrition), it was concluded that the diets of the children were as deficient in energy as they were in protein, and they needed a focus on a variety of nutrient-dense foods rather than solely concentrating on just protein. According to the FAO, the current view is that most PEM is the result of inadequate intake or poor utilization of food and energy, not deficiency of one nutrient and not usually simply a lack of dietary protein.

Even though the results of this research were clear and undeniable by the mid-1970s, the idea of protein as our supreme savior was somehow lodged deeply in Western minds. Not only did this begin a push for high-protein diets, but it specifically promoted animal foods and, later, boosted the market for protein supplements. We were introduced to terms like "complete versus incomplete proteins." These concepts, although misleading, made plant foods seem inadequate and inferior. A diet without animal products became unfathomable for most, being considered anywhere from foolish to outright dangerous. Yet despite its abundance in most foods and the extreme unlikelihood of any of us even coming close to a protein deficiency, to this day, most people in the general population harbor a very illusive fear of not getting enough protein.

The good news is that the views began to shift around the turn of the twenty-first century. We know today that there are many reasons why the focus on protein became so inflated. A big part of the problem stems from corporate and economic interests of both the animal-farming and protein supplement industries. Most of us have no idea how negatively our protein obsession works against us in so many ways: health, financial, environmental, etc. Luckily, we also have an ever-increasing number of health and nutrition experts speaking out about the dangers of high-protein diets—yes, the *dangers*! Not only that, but it has been shown over and over again that getting enough protein is not a valid concern, as long as we are eating enough food of a varied nature on a regular basis, and do not suffer from any serious health conditions that would prevent proper protein digestion or utilization. Whether we are a child or an adult, a vegan, vegetarian, athlete, or plant-based eater, getting a sufficient amount of protein is one of the easiest things to accomplish.

I presume it will still take some time to undo some of the heavy conditioning that has infiltrated into the general population regarding protein, so let's look at the specifics when it comes to the numbers. Depending on which health or nutrition expert you consult, it is likely that you will get quite a range of possible numbers. Percentage-wise, you might hear recommendations of anywhere from 5 to 50 percent of your daily calories to come from protein. The more general and commonly accepted recommendations range from 10 to 15 percent of protein from daily calories. Anything over 35 percent is considered excessive, if not, outright dangerous.

It is considered most accurate for protein requirements to be based on body weight, per pound or kilogram of our weight. Even so, there is still a wide variety of numbers, depending on the organization we consult and when. Consider the following data for further amplification of this point, protein values for adults based on organization and set time:

Organization	Recommended Protein/kg	Recommended Protein/lb
FAO/WHO (2007)	0.66g/kg	0.30g/lb
FAO/WHO (1973)	0.60g/kg	0.27g/lb
FAO/WHO (1965)	0.71g/kg	0.32g/lb
USDA and Health Canada	EAR = 0.66g/kg	EAR = 0.30g/lb
USDA and Health Canada	RDA/AI = 0.80g/kg	RDA/AI = 0.36g/lb
Fitness/Weight Training Community	AI = 1.2 - 1.4g/kg	AI = 0.55g/lb - 0.64g/lb
Fitness/Weight Training Community	UL = 1.7 - 1.8g/kg	UL = 0.77 - 0.82g/lb

Legend

EAR = Estimated Average Requirement
RDA = Recommended Dietary Allowance

AI = Adequate Intake
UL = Upper Intake Level or Upper Limit

General guidelines for amounts of daily protein in grams for women recommend that we get anywhere from 30 to 50g of protein, 40 to 60g for men. Some of us may be surprised by how little is actually recommended, based on our previous perceptions. In fact, most of us will be very surprised by how easy it is to reach or even surpass the upper limits of these ranges on a solely whole food, plant-based diet, never mind when animal products are also included. It really is unfortunate that we've bought so heavily into the ideas of not enough protein or not enough quality protein. Leafy greens alone are protein powerhouses, and they fit in perfectly with the guidelines set forth in this book. As you will recall, they are also the most powerful addition to our diet for nutrient-density and the acid-alkaline balance, thus promoting optimal health, weight, healing, and prevention.

According to the 2005-06 National Health and Nutrition Examination Survey (NHANES), both men and women ages twenty and over in the U.S. were taking in much more than the recommended amount of protein. The RDA of protein for women is 46g, and the study showed that women, on average, were taking in 70.1g. The RDA of protein for men is 56g and the results showed that, on average, men were taking in 101.9g. Both of these are nearly double the recommendations, even with the built-in safety margin. Many people learn these types of facts but still see nothing wrong with it, as there is a deeply lodged idea that the more protein, the better. However, numerous sources of research today continue to warn against high-protein, specifically high animal-protein, diets. Not only can they be a source of excess calories, but they can stress our organs and systems and lead to various imbalances in the acid-alkaline levels, our health, and weight.

In my experience with nutrition research and teaching, it has become clear that one of the main reasons why people have this peculiar insecurity about getting enough protein is that they don't know how much protein actually is in food. We may hear from sources that we should get this amount or that, but most of us do not follow up to learn how easy it is to get that amount, if that is our concern. Additionally, many people still refer to certain foods as the protein of a meal, negating the fact that there is some protein in nearly *every* food source! Not one food out there is 100 percent protein, and almost all are composed of varying amounts of each of the three macronutrients. Animal foods, which are often credited for being the protein, commonly contain either an equivalent or even a higher amount of fat than protein; it is interesting that we don't consider them the fat of a meal. Eggs and dairy are a perfect example of this if we consume them in their least processed forms, as presented below.

Food	Calories	Fat	Protein
1 Egg (whole, cooked)	77	58%	31%
1 cup Milk (whole)	146	49%	22%
1 Cheese Slice 28g (whole, cheddar, diced)	113	72%	25%

Source: nutritiondata.self.com

When considering meat for protein, including seafood it all depends on the type, source, and preparation method. Even lean meats provide varying amounts of animal fats that have been correlated with health and weight problems. Additionally, these often come with whopping amounts of calories and protein. The latter of which, as we are learning today, is not a cause for a celebration.

Food	Calories	Fat	Protein
1 Beef Steak 393g (top sirloin, separable lean and fat, trimmed to 0" fat, choice, cooked, broiled)	861	43%	53%
1 Halibut Fillet 318g (fish, Atlantic and Pacific, cooked, dry heat)	446	20%	75%
1 Chicken Breast 172g (broilers or fryers, meat only, skin removed, cooked, roasted)	284	19%	76%

Source: nutritiondata.self.com

On the other end of the spectrum are the plant foods. These not only contain protein, but also contain optimally adequate amounts of it. It is worthy to notice that their protein profiles align easily and naturally with our daily protein percentage recommendations. They also come with outstanding nutrient density profiles, as discussed in previous chapters. This means they provide a lot for a little when it comes to their nutrient:calorie ratios. They contain fiber, phytonutrients, antioxidants, and plant fats, all of which have been strongly linked with being protective, healing, and beneficial for our health and weight. Let's compare a few examples in terms of fat and protein, just as we did with the animal food sources above.

Food	Calories	Fat	Protein
1 cup Beans (kidney, all types, cooked, boiled)	225	4%	27%
1 cup Quinoa (cooked)	222	16%	14%
1 cup Brown Rice (long grain, cooked)	216	8%	9%
¼ cup Almonds (raw)	206	78%	15%
1 cup Portabella (mushrooms, grilled, sliced)	42	21%	48%
1 cup Spinach (raw)	7	12%	50%
1 cup Kale (raw, chopped)	33	18%	24%
1 cup Broccoli (raw, florettes)	20	~0%	40%
1 serving Fruits (raw, all varieties)	~50-100	~0-8%	~5-12%

Source: nutritiondata.self.com

All foods, with the exception of pure fats or sugars, contain protein, and we know today that no special combining or fussing needs to happen to get enough or the right type. All of this is easy to navigate when we take a holistic rather than reductionist approach. Nature does not provide us with nutrition labels and eating manuals. Simply eat enough food to meet your daily needs, whether it be fully from plants, or include small amounts of animal products, as outlined in Chapter 12. Choose whole foods, diversify your meals, and enjoy! Mother Nature wants you to eat and to eat well!

The protein numbers game becomes even more complex if we start to dissect how much protein we should theoretically eat per meal and before or after a physical workout. But wait, there is more! We also know that not all protein is digested or assimilated in equal ways. Proteins, like most nutrients, are heat sensitive. Heat will change their shape, structure, and/or function. We cannot overlook the fact that this may interfere with how our bodies recognize, digest, or use the altered proteins. Therefore, a lot of speculation has gone into the effects and consequences of cooked food, especially cooked animal flesh, on our health, weight, and the aging process. We covered some of this in Chapter 5. Various percentages circulate about the digestibility of various proteins from animal and plant foods, as well as their bioavailability after being subjected to typical cooking temperatures. Research is still limited in this area, but what we can conclude with certainty is that heavily heat-processed nutrients like protein are definitely not the same as their unprocessed counterparts.

It is nothing short of ironic that in our overfed, animal-food-driven societies, we even give a second thought to the possibility of not getting enough protein. Our biggest nutrition problems revolve around eating too much high-calorie and nutrient-deficient food. Of course, it doesn't help that so many health, nutrition, and fitness organizations or experts still talk about protein as if consuming it equates with guaranteed muscle mass. Some basic biology is usually omitted from the whole story here. Your body will build and maintain muscles based on its needs; it is highly dependent on the quality of your lifestyle when it comes to physical activity and the *overall* quality of your diet. Still, day after day, millions consume additional protein powders and products in the hope that these will contribute to better health and well-sculpted bodies. There is a reason our health and weight is suffering, and it isn't because we are not getting enough protein. Rather, it is because we eat too much processed and animal-based food and don't incorporate enough quality movement. This throws our bodies out of their optimal states of balance.

If you are interested in playing the protein numbers game, I simply encourage you to follow through fully. Learn about how many grams of protein are found in the servings of foods you eat regularly. You can use the following website to do so easily: nutritiondata.self.com You can do a little experiment for yourself, and keep track of your meals and drinks for a week to see how much protein you are typically consuming. Of course, if you would rather adopt a much more natural way to eat and live, I completely understand, and this is what I am hoping to inspire you to embrace through the information presented in this book. It is unnatural and unnecessary to live by nutrient numbers. Sure, they can offer guidelines, but all too often we become enslaved by those guidelines in negative ways. Not only should we avoid obsessing about numbers for optimal health, healing, and prevention, but such an obsession can add unnecessary work and stress to our lives. Connect with your body, connect with your food, and trust in the innate intelligence of nature.

Vitamins & Minerals

The story of vitamins and minerals is not very different from the macronutrients. RDAs and DRIs have been established, but as we talked about in Chapter 16, these are not uniformly accepted. What the numbers have accomplished is to give supplement-makers a marker for their formulations. For the rest of us, the numbers are either completely overlooked due to the amount of work that seems to accompany trying to understand them, or they serve as a source of stress in trying to adequately meet them. Don't get me wrong: the numbers have provided some very valuable guidance for the medical community. However, every body is unique, and none of us are robots who can be programmed to function within fixed parameters. Some days, weeks, months, and years, we need more of this and less of that. We go through various periods of vitality and stress, various life stages, and live in various geographical locations. All of these factors play a role in our health and our personal needs, and they must all be considered and addressed holistically.

As we covered in Chapter 16, we cannot let the isolated, nutrient numbers dictate whether or not we use supplements, unless we have official results from a healthcare provider and need to correct a deficiency. Instead of focusing on the numbers and isolated nutrients, focus on a nutrient-dense, richly-varied diet, choosing the best-quality, fresh, natural, whole plant foods, with an emphasis on vegetables and fruits. The healing, prevention, and weight benefits that these offer are a much better investment of your time, energy, and financial resources than trying to decipher the world of supplements. Before you invest in a multivitamin, for example, consider investing in organic foods. The synergistic effects of real, natural, whole foods are worth more than we can imagine, more than our reductionist science is able to fully grasp at this point. It is likely that, as we continue our research into phytonutrients, there will come a time where numbers will be suggested for some of those as well, but that will not necessarily make us healthier or make our lives any easier. The ways of nature are simple and efficient, not nearly as complicated as our modern world has, all too often, falsely asserted. Everything we need is packaged perfectly for us in whole, fresh plant foods. We should strive to consume these and protect them and their environments so they can continue to provide us with the best nutrients and benefits naturally.

Nutrition Facts Labels

"Instead of emphasizing one nutrient, we need to move to food-based recommendations. What we eat should be whole, minimally processed, nutritious food—food that is in many cases as close to its natural form as possible."

— Dr. Dariush Mozaffarian MD, DrPH.,
Friedman School of Nutrition, Tufts University

The final players to consider in the numbers game are the nutrition labels themselves. These are commonly found on the back or side panels of our food packages. They are typically black and white, commonly located close to the ingredients. In a sense, if we are going to follow the guidance shared in this book and make dietary choices that reflect healing and prevention, nutrition facts labels shouldn't even be of much concern to us, as they are specifically associated with processed or refined, prepackaged foods. However, given that each of us is taking this journey at our own pace, various refined foods will likely impact our lives to some degree as we continue moving in the direction of superior nutrition. These labels are also becoming commonplace at many restaurants, so being acquainted with them, at least on some level, is a good idea in today's society. Additionally, it is helpful to be aware of what I am about to share with you so that you can educate and inspire others to make wiser choices in this area.

Nutrition-labeling is a rather new phenomenon that has evolved over time and varies from country to country. Up until the late 1960s, there was little information on food labels to identify the nutrient content. Until the dawn of processed and prepackaged food, there was also little use for nutrition labels as the focus was still largely on whole, real, and unrefined foods. From around the 1960s to the late 1990s, although steps were taken to initiate nutrition-labeling, labeling in North America was voluntary. In the U.S., the 1990 Nutrition

219

Labeling and Education Act (NLEA) was passed, requiring all packaged foods to bear nutrition labels and all health claims for foods to be consistent with terms defined by the Secretary of Health and Human Services. In Canada, regulations passed in 2003 required most prepackaged foods to bear a standardized nutrition facts label; this was fully phased in by 2007. In most countries, the labels must follow a certain format and contain certain mandatory information.

As mentioned above, the necessity for this labeling was spurred by the rise of processed foods. Before then, people mainly ate wholesome foods and prepared their own meals at home, so there was little need for any such labeling. As more foods of the refined, convenience, and prepackaged nature surfaced, it became apparent that it would be a good idea to know what the foods contain, from both an ingredient and nutrient standpoint. Unfortunately, while it was an admirable idea to inform consumers about their food, this backfired, to a great degree. In this section, I will share with you some guidance for using these labels, as well as some of the major problems associated with them.

One of the saddest, most ironic things about the labels is that something intended to help us has created so much confusion about our food. It has made eating challenging, to say the least. If one is truly interested in knowing how the labels are created, how they work, and how to understand them, it actually requires some serious education on our part. There are articles, documents, books, and classes for proper understanding and use of the labels. While this could be seen as the upside to their challenging downside, I regret to inform you that even if you consult several of these resources, you will not necessarily find the same interpretations. As you already know, understanding of nutrition today varies between nutritionists, dietitians, and health professionals. The good news is that if we understand some of the basic parameters and limitations of the labels, we can actually learn a lot from them. Part of my work is to simplify things for people and help connect the dots so we can all see the bigger picture; hopefully, you are experiencing this as you read this book. This applies to nutrition facts labels as well.

For starters, we must understand that many of these labels, if not most of them, have a variable margin of error. Their accuracy truly depends on the skill and resources of the respective food company. Many simply use information from nutrition data websites, like the one I referenced earlier in this chapter, and piece together what they need. This is because it is a rather expensive process to have the food composition thoroughly and specifically analyzed in a lab. However, nutrition data sites have their own margins of error. Added to this, as we know from Chapter 6 on eating organics, nutritional value varies based on the region, soil quality, method of growing, variety of the specific food, and other factors. Also, some nutrition labels do not take into account any processing the food underwent or may undergo, which will further impact its nutrition composition. So while the labels will give us a general idea about our food, don't hold them to being 100 percent accurate. Second, areas of the label that refer to the daily value and offer percentages are related to the mainstream nutrient recommendations, like the RDA or AI. If those numbers are going to be of any use to you, you have to be in total agreement with the RDA. Generally speaking, the listed percentages can easily lead to more nutritional confusion, so I recommend that you don't ever invest your time to read them. Third, even if we are going to read the numbers, we have to have some knowledge and understanding of what is considered a so-called good or bad amount. Finally, you will still have to do some of your own math if you want a more complete story about your food. A common criticism of the labels is that they present information for servings that may not be a realistic representation of what would be consumed in a typical sitting. The servings could also be difficult to gauge, with respect as to how much is really consumed; at the very least, you will have to multiply all the numbers by the number of servings you are planning to eat. And, doing your own calculations does not only apply to servings. As I shared with you in Chapter 12, figuring out the actual percentage of fat (or any other macronutrient) that the particular food contains reveals even more valuable information.

Aside from all the issues mentioned above, if we base our dietary choices on the numbers of the nutrition facts label alone, we will miss the most important information about our food, failing to learn anything about the actual ingredients used or their quality. Remember that all fats, sugars, carbohydrates, proteins, vitamins, and minerals are not considered equal. Looking at just the nutrition facts labels, there is plenty we won't know: what kinds of sugars, sweeteners, salt, or salt enhancers are used; whether there are any possible GMO ingredients; what kinds of grains are used and if they are whole; what kinds of fats are used and if any are hydrogenated; whether there are any preservatives, artificial flavors, or colors and what kinds. I have come across too many people to date who believe they are making healthy choices simply based on the nutrition facts labels. This is a perfect example of how misleading the labels have become, as they offer anywhere from a mildly to seriously incomplete picture of our food and, hence, the quality of our nutrition. You may recall from Chapter 1 our discussion about the word healthy and the many forms it can take. This is a perfect example. If health was just about numbers like calories and nutrients, then our health and weight statistics would look a whole lot different than they do. As we know, this is simply not the case. We are not simple, static machines; we are living, dynamic beings who require the synergy and completeness of real, wholesome, quality food and nutrients.

So, is there any value to reading the labels at all? That depends on who you are, what you need, and how you understand nutrition. For those who eat highly processed diets, perhaps seeing that there are trans fats present or high values for some of the unfavorable constituents will serve as a deterrent. From my perspective, the labels are most useful for discovering the sodium level in food and possibly the macronutrient percentage when you are willing to do your own math. The daily value percentages, as I've already mentioned, are pretty much useless, as are the micronutrient percentages, which distort our understanding of the vitamin and mineral content of food. As for calories, as we covered earlier in this chapter, managing them is simply not enough to warrant good health and weight, even assuming you do the math right per food consumed and keep track of your daily totals. The value of the nutrition label is, at best, a partial overview of our food, but I would not recommend getting caught up in their number games either.

Given everything I've shared above, I hope you see that if we are interested in optimal health, healing, prevention, and weight, we are not going to find our answers on the very limited and often confusing nutrition facts labels. Yes, they can give us some idea about our food, but they provide too little of the whole story, and too much of a flawed story. If you are going to consume any processed, refined, convenience or prepackaged food, you must read the ingredients. They provide the key with which to unlock a more complete picture of your food in order to accurately assess and understand it. Above and beyond that, if you also consult the nutrition facts label, it may offer further value to make the smartest, healthiest choices for you.

Numbers Challenges

When writing this chapter, I decided to call it "The Numbers Game," since it often feels like one when we begin to delve into the world of modern nutrition and the numbers that govern it. In the last section of this chapter, I wish to bring to your attention four other areas that further limit our use of numbers in the field of nutrition.

Bioavailability

During the vast research in the field of nutrition from the mid- to late 1900s it became apparent that a simple analysis of the total concentration of a nutrient in a particular food was not a sufficient measure of its adequacy for us. Underlying factors had to be considered, mainly the notion of a nutrient's bioavailability. It may be nice to know how many grams or calories a certain nutrient is worth per serving, but this is not a fully accurate overview of what our body will actually get in the end. Numerous factors come into play here, and each one imposes various limitations on how much of a particular nutrient we will actually digest, absorb, and use. These include but are not limited to: the health of our digestive system, our overall health, the presence of any digestive inhibitors, the quality of our food, the method of food preparation, the particular combination of food consumed, and the amount of food consumed. We know, for example, that increasing the intake of one isolated mineral could result in impaired use or absorption of others. It ultimately comes back to the fact that you are a dynamic living being, not a robotic machine who will always process things the same way. The same goes for our food and its many variable properties. The nutrient values associated with a particular food or found on a food package are by no means guaranteed to be the nutrient amounts that end up in your blood, cells, tissues.

Evolving Research

The second challenge we face when it comes to the numbers in nutrition is that they are in no way constant or universally accepted. They vary, and by a lot at times! Not only do they change every few years or decades, but they also vary by geographic region on our planet. Whether it is the macro- or micronutrients, several variations exist as to what is an ideal or adequate intake. In many cases, it is impossible for experts to agree on one defined nutrition quantity, even in the same region, let alone experts or health organizations amongst different countries. This does not need to be a problem for us, as long as the numbers are used with discerning flexibility. After all, these are only generalized guidelines. However, it can become a problem when consumers and health experts latch on to the numbers conservatively, often leaving little room for questioning, margins of error, unique individual needs, or deeper introspection.

If a mainstream consumer living in North America today tries to educate themselves about the quantity of the various nutrients needed daily, they will most likely consult DRI and RDA resources. These documents provide the general, agreed-upon numbers based on various sources and research collected up to this point. However, many of these numbers are highly controversial and questioned or disputed by numerous health professionals, though the average consumer is not aware of this. In trying to be healthy, far too many eat by the numbers. This causes us to run into various challenges or problems for our health and weight, not to mention making the act of nourishment an arduous task.

Industry Collusion

Another factor that should be mentioned here is that many of the very same governing agencies that provide these numbers have very strong ties to various large industries that stand to benefit from the numbers themselves. It is no secret that top-ranking executives frequently change jobs between industries and the agencies that govern them. Personal stakes, gains, and bias must be considered here, as these will influence the outcomes for us, as consumers, to some extent. It is also no secret that large industries, like meat and dairy, have influenced public nutrition policy for decades! There is a lot of money to be gained or lost, depending on how policies and guidelines are set. While it would be great to have honest, dependable numbers, other factors aside, that are not based on any industrial or economic influences, this is simply not the case. Therefore, when it comes to the numbers, the best advice is to take them with a grain of salt.

Unique Biochemistry

The last and equally important challenge to consider when dealing with nutrition numbers is what has already been mentioned above: our unique and individual biochemistry. I will be the first to say that we have more similarities than differences when it comes to our nutrition needs as human beings. Still, there is no doubt that differences like age, sex, race, body type, weight, geographic home location, overall health, and similar factors all play a role with respect to our particular needs at any given time. We are dynamic beings who grow, change, and evolve. Different needs and stresses impact us daily and in all the various seasons of our lives.

While there are some general nutrition guidelines everyone can benefit from, as outlined in this book, problems surface when we narrow our focus too much and try to apply rigid, specific rules and numbers to everyone. For example, three middle-aged women may all be told they should get 1500mg of calcium daily by their healthcare provider. This sounds straightforward in theory, but in practice, it is not that simple. To provide each woman with the most effective advice for her, we would need to examine her diet, lifestyle habits, body type, state of health, and so on. Naturally, most practitioners or literature sources will not delve that deep, as it would require a time-consuming and perhaps costly analysis. The orthomolecular field of medicine, as well as some holistic practitioners, remain the exception, working to restore the optimum environment of the body by correcting imbalances or deficiencies based on individual biochemistry. The across-the-board number generalizations are another reason why so much nutrition confusion exists today, as many media stories simply give us a very limited scope or partial view of the complete picture.

We can most definitely appreciate the advancements that science has provided us with in the field of nutrition today, but we also have to be aware of their limitations. As we conclude this chapter, my final tip for you is to be a smart, discerning, and conscious player in the numbers game. Don't negate or ignore what we've learned thus far, but also, don't think the numbers are the say-all-that-ends-all. The numbers offer us an important glimpse, but we must fill in the rest of the picture by applying a more holistic perspective.

CHAPTER 18
Your Kitchen

One of the key determining factors for how effective we will be when it comes to optimally healthy meal preparation is the state of our kitchen. While there are many ways to make our kitchens more or less user friendly, our meal preparation habits and kitchen tools will have a tremendous impact on the level of success, quality, and enjoyment of preparing natural, wholesome, homemade meals. Basically put, we need the right tools for the right job.

Although switching over to natural, wholesome, homemade meals may mean we need to invest a little more time and money in our kitchens at first, the benefits are well worth it and will provide an ongoing return on your investment. In the long run, having the right tools and habits can save us time, increase our efficiency, and help us easily create nutritionally wholesome meals that will benefit the health, weight, and wellbeing for us and our families. In this chapter, we will examine some of these tools and habits.

Blender

One of the most fundamental tools for quick, easy, versatile, and wholesome meal preparation is a blender, but you cannot rely on just any blender. Specifically, you will benefit the most from a high-powered, commercial-grade blender. Two of the most common choices are Vitamix and Blendtec. These will literally transform your meals and improve meal preparation time. If you have experience with an ordinary blender and/or have never heard of these brands, you will naturally wonder what makes them stand out, aside from their price tag. As these units typically cost three to five times more than a typical blender, it is only natural to question their value. At first glimpse, I also found it difficult to justify their cost. After all, what could possibly be so special about a blender? I began my journey with an ordinary Black & Decker blender, and at the time, it seemed to meet my needs relatively well. Little did I know what was possible!

After seeing a Vitamix demo at a home show, I was in disbelief at the power of the machine. Whatever food you can imagine, down to the tiniest seed, it will pulverize into the smoothest, finest consistency! That day, I vowed that I would make owning one a priority in my life. At the start of 2010, that intention became a reality, and I became the proud owner of a Vitamix. Aside from when I travel, I don't think a day has passed when I haven't put it to use; in fact, I often use it two or three times a day. My kitchen and meals wouldn't be the same without it, as it completely transformed my meals thanks to its power, versatility, and capability. After several years, one gets so used to it that it is easy to forget that this is not the norm for all blenders. Luckily, during some travels, I had the chance to try some ordinary blenders and was quickly reminded of the unmistakable difference. If you haven't guessed already, I am an avid fan of green smoothies; my mornings wouldn't be the same without them. Thanks to my Vitamix, I can create amazing combinations with no leaf, vegetable, fruit, nut, or seed pieces or parts left to chew. It provides an amazing, uniformly smooth final product, and this plays an integral role in optimally healthy eating, as we must enjoy the flavor and consistency of our food if we are going to have a chance at making it work for us.

Whether you get a Vitamix or Blendtec is up to you. Research them both and see what features suit your personal preferences. Most importantly, watch a demo, in person or in a video online. These blenders are able to pulverize or grind any food finely, and they can also chop, dice, or juice, all in a matter of seconds or minutes. You can quickly and easily make fresh, wholesome smoothies, juices, non-dairy milks, purées, soups, nut butters, bean spreads, dips, sauces, dressings, pestos, non-dairy ice cream, and so much more, and cleanup is super quick and easy as well. For all these reasons, I highly recommend them as an essential part of any kitchen for optimally healthy meal preparation that is ultra quick, simple, and enjoyable.

Food Processor

A food processor is also a great addition to your kitchen, but it is not a necessity, especially if you own one of the blenders mentioned above. Whether or not you need one depends on your family's needs or your personal meal preferences. For example, it may be more efficient to hand-chop vegetables for a salad for one or two people. However, if you are making a salad for a family of four or more, a food processor would be much more efficient and practical. There may also be some meal or snack ideas that would be best made using a food processor. The snacks and desserts listed in the meal ideas of Chapter 15 are a good example. I always use my food processor to make them, as opposed to my Vitamix.

When it comes to food processors, I have not found as many differences between the low- and high-end models as with the blenders. I once owned a simple Black & Decker, but today I use a high-performance Cuisinart model. While there are some obvious benefits to a higher-end model, any well-reviewed, powerful enough, user-friendly food processor should be suitable. In your search, look for something that is durable. Many units today are constructed with a lot of plastic parts, and these can easily crack or break during normal use.

Juicer

Another common kitchen tool that is often equated with optimal health and weight is a juicer. Although these have been around for decades, the practice of juicing has grown significantly in popularity during the last few years alone: from Jay Kordich, the Father of Juicing, whose personal cancer-healing journey in 1948 was assisted by the late Dr. Max Gerson, to Joe Cross and his 2010 film, *Fat, Sick & Nearly Dead*, where he went on a 60-day juice fast to lose 100 pounds and heal his body. Juicing can be used for various health, healing, and prevention purposes, which we will discuss in the next chapter. For now, let's focus on how to pick the best juicer.

When it comes to juicers, there are two main kinds: centrifugal and masticating. How they operate, how well they juice, how easy they are to clean, how much countertop space they take up, and how much they cost depends heavily on the kind you get. Centrifugal juicers tend to be cheaper and easier to clean, but they are usually not as good at extracting juice or maintaining the nutritional integrity of the juice. Masticating juicers tend to offer excellent juice yield and quality, but are normally more complex, timely to use, and costly. Your choice depends on how you plan to approach your juicing journey, as well as any personal preferences or limitations. Either way, it is essential to undertake thorough research when it comes to choosing a juicer. The right one will make a world of a difference in every way possible, from the quality of the final product to how often you end up using it.

In your decision, consider your lifestyle as well. If you are constantly on the go or have young children who require much of your time, a masticating juicer may not be a very practical choice for you. If you want to juice lots of leafy greens, including wheat grass, a centrifugal juicer may not be the best option. As for the price tag, a cheaper juicer may be enticing, but consider how much money you will be wasting on a regular basis if it is not efficient at extracting juice from your produce. Read up and research your juicer properly before committing and making a purchase. Most popular, high-rated juicers come from brands like Green Star, Kuvings, Omega, and Breville.

Dehydrator

In understanding the value of raw foods, many people begin to explore dehydrators. These units can process and preserve your foods at low temperatures without destroying their nutritional integrity, similar to the way an oven would but without exposing the food to damaging heat. Dehydrators are excellent if you are interested in making truly raw versions of your own dried fruits, vegetables, herbs, granola, crackers, pizza crusts, various bars, desserts, healthy pet treats, and more.

A dehydrator can be a costly investment, and while it can be very beneficial, it is certainly not essential. It is one of those tools I typically recommend for people who have already gone well into their journey of optimal health, healing, and prevention, though there are exceptions, and some people make them a top priority at the start of their healthy eating journey. Again, it all depends on your personal lifestyle, preferences, priorities, finances, and kitchen space.

Dehydrators typically take up a good chunk of your counter space, so be sure to factor that in, unless you have another space where you plan to store it for regular use. A home dehydrator will typically cost anywhere from $200 to $500, depending on the size you choose. Aside from providing optimal nutrition choices, dehydrators are also a very popular choice amongst those who like to be more self-sufficient and preserve their own food. The most common, trusted name in dehydrators is Excalibur.

Sprouter

As we've talked about in our nut, seed, grain, and bean chapters, sprouts are some of the most beneficial foods for our health, weight, healing, and prevention. While it is possible to purchase some sprouts these days at your local grocery store or farmers' market, an increasing number of people are choosing to sprout at home. Sprouting can be a fairly simple, straightforward process, but it does require some time and incorporation into your daily routine. This is where a sprouter can help.

When I first began sprouting, I simply used a plate, paper towel, and lid. This was very simple but was not overly practical. Many people use reusable glass jars or various trays and create their own homemade sprouters. One of the best methods for sprouting is a glass jar with a screen lid. This is also the most cost-effective way to go. Sprouters can be purchased, but they are usually just very simple plastic or glass units. While they are relatively inexpensive, they still may not be necessary, since you can accomplish your own sprouting with a simple glass jar. There are numerous videos and articles available online today that demonstrate the process and provide tips for the different foods to be sprouted.

Toaster Oven

Although we want to maintain the nutritional integrity of our food as much as possible and consume it in its natural, fresh, raw forms, there are times when cooked foods are welcome and even necessary. Stovetop cooking, like steaming and sautéing, are, perhaps, the best ways to gently heat-process our food. Cooking potatoes, soup, beans, or some grains can make them more palatable. What we want to avoid, as we talked about in Chapter 5, is exposing our foods to high, prolonged, and/or destructive heat, like frying, or grilling. As such, you will not use your oven very much, if at all. A toaster oven, however, can come in handy. Whether you wish to cook some portobello mushrooms or gently warm something, this can be an efficient choice rather than using the resources required by a standard-sized oven.

Other Tools & Gadgets

It is always a good idea to have a basic peeler. This is especially useful for times when you may not be able to find organic versions of your produce. Removing the skin from cucumbers or apples can lessen the pesticide load, at least to some extent.

You will work with lemons a lot for the various salads, soups, dressings, and such, so it helps to have a lemon squeezer, reamer, or press, as well as a small sieve or strainer. You can choose from plastic, glass, wood, or metal devices, but it is a wise idea to use as little plastic as possible, and I would also recommend staying away from metal, due to the initial acidic nature of citrus. Whatever you choose, the trick to getting the most juice out of your fresh lemons is to roll them several times on a hard surface, like your cutting board, applying some pressure with the rolling hand, then cut them open and squeeze accordingly.

One of my favorite tools that I use with my Vitamix blender and food processor is a spatula. This versatile tool constantly comes in handy for many daily uses. Aside from the fact that I do not like to waste any food, an ideal I encourage, a spatula is the best way to fully remove the contents from your blender, food processor, pot, or dish. It can also be used to pat down or spread ingredients during the making of your optimally healthy desserts, like those I shared with you in Chapter 15.

Although the idea is to get comfortable in working with whole, natural plant food, to the extent that you won't need to rely on specific measurements or recipes, a measuring cup is a must-have. Let's face it: Sometimes precise measurements can make or break a successful meal preparation. For example, something as simple as cooking brown rice can be a triumphant endeavor if you measure the right amount of water for the rice you are cooking. Whether for general grain and bean cooking or for some special, specific recipe, it is really worth having a good measuring cup handy. In terms of quality, make sure your measuring cup is made of glass, not plastic. The most versatile is a two-cup size, which should meet all your needs easily.

Since you will be working with a lot of fresh vegetables, mushrooms, and fruits, a good knife and cutting board are essential. Some people wish to have several quality knives of different sizes, but I personally prefer one versatile, good knife for all of my meal preparation. I do have a knife block with a few different sizes, but I rarely use any of them. Most importantly, to easily chop and dice your vegetables, mushrooms and fruits, make sure your knife is very sharp, as this will make the process that much smoother. In terms of a cutting board, the size and shape is completely up to you. I only recommend glass or wood, such as bamboo, and it is best to avoid plastic ones. Keep in mind that if you eat animal products, you should have a separate cutting board for them and cut your plant foods on one strictly intended for them so as to avoid cross-contamination.

When it comes to cookware, the choices are many and not often easy. There is a wide range of prices and materials, like stainless steel, cast iron, copper, and ceramic. Nonstick cookware should not be an option in an optimally healthy home, as we will discuss in the next section. Aluminum cookware should also be avoided, due to its risk of toxicity. For most people, copper cookware is just fine, but be aware that a small percentage of the population may be at increased risk to copper toxicity, especially if you cook a lot of acidic substances regularly. Ceramic and clay options used to be a good idea, before we unleashed all sorts of chemical paints, varnishes, and coatings on them. Thus, the best options really come down to stainless steel and cast iron. Stainless steel is most versatile and affordable and, as far as we know, least problematic. Cast iron is an extremely healthy choice for most, except for those in the population who are at risk to iron overload. If choosing cast iron, be sure to buy real cast iron and properly season it yourself; do not use those coated with novel materials of questionable safety. A typical eight- to twelve-piece set should meet most of your needs. When shopping for a new set, pay extra attention to the handles, as these are often one of the most important features to make your cooking safe and enjoyable, as well as the lids. Some handles heat up and require oven mitts for handling, and others are flimsy or awkward, especially when the pot is full and heavy. With respect to lids, I personally love see-through lids, since they can help you gauge the readiness of your food and avoid over-steaming vegetables or undercooking grains. Cookware can range in price based on various factors. Research your options, depending on your budget and cooking needs.

In terms of bakeware, the assumption on the path to optimal nutrition is that you will do little baking, if any at all. In any case, glass bakeware is a better option than any kind of nonstick. You should easily be able to find square, rectangular, and round glass bakeware in many sizes. It is also possible to find more glassware today, made in Europe, Italy, or the United States, which may ensure an even higher product quality. Silicone bakeware is becoming increasingly popular, but lots of cheaply made options exist, and these are typically teeming with various chemicals; simply removing it from its package will assault your nostrils with the strong off-gassing of chemical odors. However, silicone can be very versatile and easy to use, thanks to its nonstick features and stain resistance. It is especially useful if you make unique, healthy treats, like homemade chocolates or truffles. Silicone is believed to have low toxicity and thermal stability, but many feel it has not been thoroughly tested yet. If silicone is something you are considering, I recommend that you use it for raw, not baked food items, only buy from reputable brands, and avoid damaging the material with any sharp objects.

In terms of food storage, it is a good idea to replace your plastic containers with glass. Today, numerous options of nearly every size and shape exist, and glass is the safest way to store our food for any period of time. And as mentioned above, you may easily find quality glassware that was manufactured in our own country. If you do choose to use any kind of plastic containers, be mindful not to put hot food in them, store them in hot areas, or cut into them with sharp objects.

There are, of course, a whole plethora of other gadgets and kitchen accessories that can be included to optimize and simplify your meal preparation, from garlic presses to salad spinners and everything in between. My advice for you here is two-fold: definitely explore the possible options that can improve your meal preparation experience, and choose what you feel would really work best for you, but err on the side of minimalism. All too often, our drawers and cupboards are filled with tools that initially seemed like a good idea but now just take up space. There are specific tools for almost any job, like grapefruit- or salad-specific knives, but do you really need it when a normal, sharp knife will do? That is a question for you to answer, based on your needs and preferences. Whatever tool or gadget you choose, be sure to pick the healthiest, least toxic options, being mindful of the material they are made of and where they are manufactured.

Things to Avoid in Your Kitchen

As you decide to add new appliances and tools to your kitchen, you will most likely benefit from making new room for them. One of the best ways to optimize kitchen space, especially if you don't have much of it, is to remove things that are not often used or things that do not contribute to healthy habits. I have three main suggestions that will ultimately make a big difference in your personal eating habits and, thus, your overall health: microwave, coffeemaker, and nonstick cookware.

Removal of the microwave should be an obvious choice if you are making a serious commitment to seek optimal heath and weight. First, the health effects are a serious concern, both in using the microwave and consuming microwaved food. You can find a plethora of information about this from many credible sources online. Of course, it may already be obvious to you when you consider the nature of how microwaves work; they actually change the molecular structure of food. In essence, using a microwave defeats the purpose of putting effort into sourcing fresh, natural, organic food. From a practical perspective, it leaves you with a big and tempting loophole to deviate from optimally healthy meal preparation. Let's face it: As long as that microwave is present, you may come home tired or find yourself in a rush and be tempted to revert to old habits. If the unit is not there, you can still put together a whole-meal smoothie in only a few minutes, and it will be much more beneficial to actually support your mind and body when you are run down. We often forget, too, that any leftovers can be easily re-warmed on the stovetop in just a few minutes. It is also worthy to consider that chopping and preparing food can actually be a tension reliever, a positive, meditative-like activity that can provide a pleasant transition and relaxation after a long or stressful day.

Another kitchen appliance you should consider parting ways with is your coffeemaker. When we eat fresh, natural, wholesome, plant-based we will automatically boost our energy level. The more we include other healthy lifestyle habits, like proper sleep and exercise, the further this benefits our vitality. The cyclical effect of eating better is that we tend to sleep better, have less cravings, and feel better, among many other positive effects. It is also easier to break our reliance on external stimulants. If you enjoy a high-quality, natural, organic cup of coffee as an occasional indulgence, it is no problem; however, most people who own coffeemakers suffer from a full-blown addiction or unconscious reliance on this substance. As already shared in Chapter 14, there is no denying that coffee may have some positive benefits, but given our high-stress lifestyles, poor diets, and coffee consumption habits, its use is to our disadvantage.

Like with the microwave, thinking of letting go of this appliance may create some anxiety. However, you will be amazed at just how fast you will adapt and adjust to a new way of living when the option to stray is no longer available. Swap your coffeemaker for a juicer, and turn a disadvantageous morning habit into a beneficial one. A fresh glass of green juice has very invigorating and nourishing properties that can offer an excellent start to your day. Plus, the more we remove processed foods and stimulants from our diet, the more we benefit our mental, emotional, and psychological health. In the end, nothing beats a naturally sharp, calm, conscious mind with which to navigate through your day.

Nonstick cookware has been a notorious topic, especially over the last two decades. By now, most health-conscious individuals are aware of the blatant dangers of using Teflon cookware, but this is not the only culprit; also consider other nonstick materials, like Silverstone, Tefal, Anolon, Circulon, Caphalon, Thermolon, and others. Most nonstick cookware contains *perfluorochemicals* like *perfluorooctanoic* acid (PFOA) and *polytetrafluoroethylene* (PTFE). These chemicals are considered toxic, are associated with serious health effects, and are suspected carcinogens. Although passed as "safe under normal use," most nonstick pans get too hot in our day-to-day cooking, releasing PFOA and other toxic substances. When the Environmental Working Group (EWG) performed commissioned tests in 2003 on nonstick coated pans, they found that the pans reach temperatures that produce toxins in less than five minutes on a typical household stove.[1] Due to the fact that products such as pots and pans do not require any kind of official ingredient labels like food or personal care products do, we can never be really sure of what is in them. Some new, nonstick technology cookware, like Thermolon, does not contain perfluorochemicals like PFOA or PTFE, but we don't know for certain how these materials will fare in the long run. On top of all this, from a practical usability standpoint, my personal experience with such cookware had resulted in longer cooking time and less-than-ideal meals. Compared to a typical stainless steel pan, nonstick cookware just doesn't seem to cook foods in the right way when it comes to texture or consistency. We usually don't notice this until we try another type of cookware. Ultimately, if you do choose to use any nonstick cookware, be sure not to puncture or scratch the coating material with sharp utensils.

It is unfortunate that the whole food-sticking issue has been blown so out of proportion; it is simply not the problem it has been made out to be. It is one thing if you only have one nonstick skillet that you use properly and infrequently, on low heat only and for short cooking durations, but it is quite another if all your regularly used pots and pans are nonstick. Properly cooked grains, beans, soups, and the like never require nonstick pots. You can also easily sauté or steam mushrooms or any kind of vegetables on a regular, stainless steel skillet without any problems, whether using a little bit of water, virgin coconut oil, or neither; when covered, most vegetables and mushrooms easily produce their own juices. As long as there is some constant moisture in the pan/skillet, you should have no messy problems with sticking. Additionally, although we want to minimize our use of oils and only use heat-stable ones like virgin coconut oil if we do at all, properly preheated oil, on a low setting, will prevent sticking. As your personal needs may dictate, cast iron pans can also provide naturally nonstick surfaces. There are many choices that can work for us without relying on nonstick cookware. The bulk of it really comes down to being mindful in the kitchen and setting timers, as we will discuss below, to prevent leaving things on the stove for too long or burning them. We have many options to minimize the amount of toxins in our lives, but we must put those choices into intelligent practice.

Practical Tips for Smart Kitchen Habits

Aside from having the right tools, paying attention to some of your personal kitchen and meal preparation habits can bring further success, pleasure, and empowerment on your healthy eating journey. Here are a few tips to help:

1. **Start with a clean workspace.** Some of us use our kitchens as home administrative centers, with mail, keys, flyers, and all sorts of things piled on the countertops. There is a huge benefit, though, to a clean, uncluttered

environment, regardless of which room we are talking about. It promotes better clarity of the mind, creativity, and ease. While you are cooking, you shouldn't be thinking about the bills you need to pay; rather, focus on nourishing your body in the best of ways. A sink full of dirty dishes, food wrappers, and items that need to be put away distracts us from a good work flow. It can also make meal preparation stressful, tedious, and frustrating if you have to fight for counter space, try to find that spatula at the bottom of the dirty dish pile, or stave off anxiety about all that needs to get done. This tip goes hand in hand with Tip 7; once you get into a good routine, these will naturally sponsor each other.

2. **Get organized.** Food preparation will take much longer and be far more frustrating if you have to invest a lot of time in finding the right tools and ingredients. Take an hour, a day, or however long you need to organize your kitchen so you know what you have and where it all is. If you live with others, try to involve them in the process and explain the benefits of keeping things organized for everyone's pleasure and convenience. This is a good time to get rid of things that may not be useful to you anymore. Once you get into the swing of your meal preparation patterns, simply be sure to put things back where they belong to maintain an organized, easy, flowing routine.

3. **Get into a mindful zone.** Meal preparation can be one of the most relaxing, meditative activities, and it will allow you to consciously connect with your food and senses. It can also be invigorating, uplifting, and exciting. Of course, this all depends on how you approach it or choose to perceive it. Rather than feeling like it is a dreaded chore, mindfully connect with your food and experience the textures, flavors, and scents as you prepare it. Consider where it came from and send gratitude to the person who grew and harvested it, even if that is you! Your mind will naturally try to ponder all sorts of other things that are part of your life, but mindfully guide yourself back to the present moment. The benefits of this are manifold. You are less likely to hurt yourself or create an unsafe situation. You are less likely to ruin the food or destroy the meal. You are more likely to enjoy yourself and learn what works and what doesn't for you for next time.

4. **Be filled with positive intentions.** Food made with love just tastes better! Most of us have experienced this firsthand at some point in our lives, and quantum science regularly emphasizes the power of thoughts and intentions on everything around us. Psychologists from the University of Maryland also performed tests that showed that good intentions can soothe pain, increase pleasure, and improve taste.[2] So, whether you are cooking for yourself, your partner, family, or friends, aside from being mindful, prepare your meals with a positive mindset and intentions: love, joy, and gratitude. Good intentions really do go a long way!

5. **Be efficient.** If you are cooking brown rice or beans, most of which take about forty-five minutes, know that there are many ways to use that time efficiently. You don't have to wait till those items are cooked before you begin chopping or steaming your vegetables. You can continue with other meal preparation during that time, or, if nothing else is needed, that time is yours to do other things nearby. You do not have to stir these items or watch over them, as long as they are on low, simmering heat and covered. Just be sure to follow Tip 6, turn on the timer, and let the cooking take care of itself. If you are preparing one of the vegetable medley mixes I talked about in Chapter 15, begin washing and chopping the longest-cooking items first and start cooking them while you continue with the prep work of the shorter-cooking items, rather than doing all your prep work beforehand. Finally, keep in mind some general meal preparation times. If you are limited on time or have a houseful of hungry mouths, it is not a good idea to make a brown rice-based dish. Choose quinoa or potatoes instead, which will typically cook in ten to fifteen minutes.

6. **Use timers.** One of the easiest ways to avoid overcooked or burned food or fire hazards on the stove is with the help of a timer. Whether you use your stove timer, a manual timer, or your Smartphone timer, use it effectively. This is one of the best and easiest ways to keep on track, stay mindful, and avoid unpleasant surprises.

7. **Finish with a clean workspace.** One of the best habits to get into is cleaning your food preparation workspace, either during the meal-making process or after the meal, along with the dishes. Choose what works best for you

and your family routine, but I cannot overemphasize the benefits of cleaning up after each meal to have quick, enjoyable, successful meal preparations, not to mention peace of mind. This will typically take only a few minutes, but it will make a world of a difference when you don't have to walk into a dirty kitchen the next time you need to make food. Making this part of every meal preparation is the easiest way to go. Of course, it goes without saying, the more mindful and efficient you are during meal prep, the less you will have to clean up later.

CHAPTER 19
Healthy Lifestyle Habits

Our food is very influential on our health, weight, and wellbeing. How you eat, what you eat, and what you don't eat each play a role in working toward or against your body's natural state of balance. While many other lifestyle areas, like sleep and exercise, are essential for consideration when it comes to the creation and maintenance of optimal health and weight, nutrition plays one of the most vital roles, second only to the power of the mind, which we will discuss in Chapter 20. Diet influences sleep quality; healthy diets are correlated with good sleep and vice versa. So, aside from healthy stress management, one of the first places to start with to improve your sleep quality for better healing and restorative effects is your diet.

When it comes to exercise, diet trumps its effects for both health and weight benefits. Please do not get me wrong: Both diet and exercise are essential components of optimal health, but more, faster, and sustainable health and weight results are achieved via diet than exercise. These are the findings and recommendations of many medical and holistic health experts alike. For example, eating less is more effective for losing weight than exercising without changing one's diet. A 2012 study published in the research journal, *Obesity*, found 8.5 percent weight loss among women who were in the diet-only group, versus 2.4 percent weight loss among those in the exercise-only group.[1] Naturally, the best results were found in those who dieted and exercised, as they came in at 10.4 percent of weight loss. One of the problems with focusing on exercise alone is that many people have the idea that they can eat whatever they want and simply work it off. Your body may respond well to burning excess calories, but health just does not work that way, as we covered in Chapter 17. In fact, an article published in the *Psychological Science* journal examined a series of studies across five countries on three continents and found that people who mainly believed obesity is caused by a lack of exercise were more likely to be overweight than those who believed it is caused by a poor diet.[2] As we will cover in Chapter 20, our thoughts and beliefs are very powerful and can easily work against us if we are not mindful or do not have the full scope of information needed to make a sound conclusion. Health is not composed of calories; it needs the right nutrients and constructive elements, while keeping out toxins and destructive elements. If weight loss or maintenance is your goal and you focus on exercise alone, you may achieve a fit body, but that doesn't guarantee it will be a healthy one. Hence, we continue to return to the multifactorial nature of health and disease that I introduced at the start of this book.

Back to my initial point, the quality of your diet will be one of the most consequential components in the creation of your present and future health, weight, and wellbeing. You can explore resource upon resource and hear from expert upon expert to gain a more detailed understanding of the diet connection to every disease condition, depending on your needs or interests. For our purposes, I hope you have, thus far, gained a thorough understanding of how to make your diet work for your optimal wellbeing, but we will not stop with diet. The whole point of taking a holistic approach to health, healing, and prevention is exploring how other internal and external factors influence our health and wellbeing. Whether it is good health, weight, detox, or even better relationships that we seek, we must give these daily focus. These goals must become part of your lifestyle, not handled as isolated events. Thus, in this chapter, I will provide you with a short, concise summary of other habits and areas of your life that require your regular, conscious attention to ensure your present and future health and wellbeing.

Green Juicing

In the previous chapter, we talked about some tools and appliances that can support our approach to optimal health. One is a juicer, and I want to briefly touch upon the benefits. Juicing is the extraction of fresh juice from a food, most notably fruits and vegetables. Its composition mainly includes water, vitamins, minerals, antioxidants, phytonutrients, and possibly some macronutrients. These juices, even if they don't contain greens, are often referred to as "green juices," so as to prevent confusion with the conventional understanding of juices: processed, pasteurized, prepackaged, empty-calorie beverages. I also like to refer to them as "living juices." What sets these juices apart from other healthy fruit and vegetable beverages, like smoothies, which we will talk about next, is that they are devoid of fiber. You are correct in questioning whether or not this is a good thing, since we know fiber is such a beneficial part of our diet. The nature of a green juice, along with the absence of fiber, makes it a readily available source of vital nutrients that our bodies easily absorb. It gives our digestive system a break, so to speak, while delivering highly digestible nutrients. This is one of the main reasons why green juices are correlated with being highly healing. They are also alkalizing, cleansing, and detoxifying.

In our daily diet, we most definitely want fiber. Generally speaking, we benefit from lots of it, but there are times when a living juice will be a welcome addition to your diet. You can enjoy such a juice daily or weekly or engage in seasonal juice fasts that last anywhere from twenty-four hours to several days. Australian filmmaker and entrepreneur Joe Cross, creator of *Fat, Sick & Nearly Dead*, chronicled his 60-day juice fast, which allowed him to shed 100 pounds and heal a slew of health conditions. If you are going to engage in strictly juicing for a few days or longer, you need to learn what to expect and how to do it in the healthiest of ways, especially if you already have an underlying health condition. To maintain the nutritional integrity of the juice and prevent it from becoming oxidized (nutritionally degraded), the right juicer will make a big difference, as we discussed in the previous chapter.

Aside from weight loss, people report all sorts of noticeable benefits from regular juicing. You won't find these covered in scientific studies yet though. If you need proof, your best bet is personal experience. Give it an honest try and see how your body responds. Reported or associated health benefits of juicing include: increased and balanced energy, stamina, and vitality; improved and/or cleared-up skin conditions; improved digestion; improved immunity; improved memory, focus, and clarity; reduced menstrual problems; and reduced cravings. Green juice positively supports the health of all of our organs and can easily be attributed with the prevention of most chronic conditions like cancer, heart disease, and diabetes. In fact, the Gerson Therapy for chronic disease healing, founded by the late Dr. Max Gerson, is based on juicing. When it comes to the famous green juice detoxing benefits, both fruits and vegetables naturally offer such support, whether in whole or juiced form, fruits tend to be more cleansing for our bodies and vegetables more detoxifying.

To make a true, optimally healthy green juice, there are a few guidelines to follow. The main premise is that the juice should be highly vegetable-based. Common ratios for most healing, prevention, and weight loss recommend an 80:20 ratio of vegetables to fruits. For example, juice a bunch of celery and one apple, or a cucumber, some ginger, and a lemon. If we get into making or solely consuming fruit or fruit-based juices, even though they are homemade and much healthier than their processed and pasteurized counterparts, they will be a higher source of calories and sugars. Green juices are most commonly and perhaps best used as snacks, when consumed outside of a juice fast, as part of your regular diet. Some people swap a meal sometimes for a large portion (16 to 32 ounces, or ½ to 1 liter) of green juice, especially if weight loss is a desired goal. If juicing is something that resonates with you or that you would like to incorporate as part of your optimally healthy lifestyle, I encourage you to explore more about this topic. Enjoy the rich variety of flavor combinations of green juices to delight your senses as you nourish your body with supportive and healing nutrients.

Green Smoothies

More common than juicing for people who embrace an optimally healthy lifestyle is blending, making smoothies. Unlike juices, which are extracts of the fruits and vegetables, smoothies incorporate the whole fruit and vegetable and their many outstanding nutrition qualities, along with the fiber. Like juices, smoothies can be used as snacks but are most often incorporated as whole meals. They are very filling, satisfying, and depending on the whole, plant food ingredients used, can provide a rich abundance of healthy fats, protein, and carbohydrates. Of course, because smoothies are based on fruits and vegetables, they're also an outstanding source of phytonutrients, antioxidants, vitamins, and minerals for our unique healing and prevention needs.

There are all sorts of smoothies, whether homemade or commercially made. It is very important to understand before we go any further that a smoothie label does not automatically qualify the beverage as healthy. In fact, many smoothies are based on processed foods, animal foods, or sugars. These are not the kinds of smoothies or blending experiences we are talking about here. To be optimal for healing and prevention, as with juices, they must be based on fresh, whole, plant foods: fruits and vegetables, specifically leafy greens. Hence, we refer to them as "green smoothies." My personal favorite way to start my day is with a green smoothie. This serves as my breakfast, gently breaks the natural fast from the night, and supplies me with top-quality nutrients in an easily digestible form. It is also my favorite and easiest way to eat my greens for breakfast! If you have never had the pleasure of trying a green smoothie, thoughts of repulsive flavors, odd textures, and off-putting colors may be running through your mind. However, I can assure you that when done right, a green smoothie can be an incredibly delicious experience. The colors are shades of vibrant and beautiful greens, unless you add in berries, which will turn them olive or purple. As for the texture, this is where the right blender will either make or break your smoothie experience; I would personally not be such a big green smoothie fan if not for my Vitamix blender. I've had green smoothies from other blenders and definitely did not enjoy chewing the various leaf pieces or other ingredients via every other sip, but I know others who actually love texture in their green smoothies. To each his or her own!

Just like with juices, the health benefits of green smoothies are many and will be best experienced based on your personal health and weight needs. Green smoothies are highly alkalizing, cleansing, and detoxifying. They can easily aid weight loss, healing, and prevention. They promote healthy elimination and digestive health. By supplying top-quality, vital nutrients, they support the body's natural balance, allowing our bodies to thrive. From your liver to your immune system, they can enhance the function of nearly every organ and system thanks to their outstanding nutrient-density. In fact, they have many of the same benefits attributed to them as the green juices above. The main difference is in the process of digestion and how fast or efficiently your body can get at those nutrients. Juicing supplies the fastest route, but smoothies come in second, as the fiber content and digestion required delays nutrient absorption. Their benefits and healing power, though, do not come as much from the fact that they are in a blended form; rather, it is because they are based on leafy greens and high concentrations of beneficial nutrients. This is where the most power lies for all our health needs. While your green smoothies can include various plant food ingredients, make sure that, first and foremost, they contain a lot of leafy greens. Review Chapter 15 for ingredient ideas and recommendations for delicious and, filling green smoothies. Additionally, you can visit my website (www.evitaochel.com) where you will find an entire video course dedicated to understanding and making optimally healthy and delicious green smoothies.

Ultimately, not everyone will be a fan of green juices and/or smoothies, and this does not only relate to personal meal preference. Some medical or nutrition experts support one and not the other. There is no need to be discouraged or confused if you come across this; remember that everyone has his or her own personal understanding of what healthy looks like. What I can guarantee is that no one will argue about the optimal benefits of fruits and vegetables, regardless of how they are consumed: whole, juiced, or blended. For ease of application and your sanity, let the similarities, rather than the differences, guide your choices.

Exercise

The benefits of exercise are as commonly known as those of healthy eating. In order to have optimal health and wellbeing we must be active. Our sedentary lifestyles are destroying our health and quality of life, literally killing us. We have countless sources of research linking exercise with good cardiovascular health. The American Heart Association outlines that a sedentary lifestyle is one of the five major risk factors (along with high blood pressure, abnormal values for blood lipids, smoking, and obesity) for cardiovascular disease.[3] There are many other benefits of exercise too. These include, but are not limited to: improving sleep; improving immune function; decreasing risk of Type 2 diabetes; decreasing risk of weight problems; reducing and/or maintaining healthy cholesterol; improving digestion and elimination; improving flexibility, stamina, balance, coordination, and endurance; reducing stress and anxiety; and numerous benefits for our mental and emotional health.[4] If your physical movement includes sweating, you can add some of the most effective detoxification benefits to that list as well. When regular exercise is coupled with an optimally healthy diet, the two provide a powerful combination that further enhances healing, prevention, and optimal health.

If the idea of exercise turns you off, replace that word with movement. Our bodies were designed to move, but staying active does not need to mean getting a membership at a gym. There are many ways to stay active naturally. Remember that our ancestors did not have Pilates, spinning class, fancy gyms, or personal trainers. What they did have was plenty of time in nature, outdoor work, and no technological devices to keep them glued to their chairs. Today, our lifestyles can be very problematic if left unchecked. First, we don't spend enough time in nature, never mind being active outdoors. Second, the great majority of us have traded in manual outdoor labor for none or automated labor. Third, we have a plethora of electronic gadgets today that entice us with video games, apps, visual entertainment, and every online service we can imagine, not to mention work that requires us to move nothing more than our fingers. These things don't need to be negative in and of themselves, but they have become harmful for our health since we have lost complete balance with respect to them. What this means for us is as follows: While our ancestors never had to give a second thought to moving enough, we do. We have to work much harder at maintaining balance in the area of physical activity, due to the nature of our lifestyles. As with everything else in life, you can make this as enjoyable or as difficult as you'd like. If you are interested in optimal health, I recommend viewing it as enjoyable. To do so, start by picking from activities you enjoy. If you like swimming, get a membership at your local pool. If you like karate, find class options that suit your schedule. If you like soccer, join a local team. Whatever you choose, a daily walk of some sort is pretty much essential. You can kayak in the summer and ski in the winter, but regardless of the season, a walk should be incorporated as part of your regular lifestyle. Whether it is ten minutes, thirty minutes, or an hour, just do it!

As with food, too much exercise can also be too much of a good thing. Although exercise is commonly equated with being a healthy habit and the majority of us are not getting enough, some have swung the pendulum in the opposite direction. Some people are actually addicted to exercise, and just like any other addiction, this can be harmful. The natural high we get from a good workout can be highly enlivening, but there are ways of doing it in safe, balanced ways. Frequent, strenuous exercise can easily wear out and wear down the body. Just ask any professional athlete or avid runner. Unnatural stress on our joints, accelerated bodily wear and tear, exaggerated pressure on our ankles and knees, as well as inflammation of overused parts are amongst the most common problems associated with overexerting ourselves. Some physical stress is good, but too much is not. Listen to your body and honor its needs appropriately. Remember that we are trying to support healing and prevention for optimal health and wellbeing, so we need to make sure we use exercise in helpful, rather than harmful ways. Anyone who has ever pushed too hard and too quickly knows the uncomfortable and even excruciating pain that can come with lactic acid buildup. As you might imagine, this causes a highly acidic state in our bodies, putting a strain on our acid-alkaline balance and, in turn, on our overall health. This may not be a big deal once in a while, especially given a properly balanced acid-alkaline diet, but if it becomes a regular occurrence, it can easily put us at increased risk for other problems. This is why we cannot look at the friend or co-worker who runs umpteen miles each day and automatically assume they are healthy. Health and healthy habits, as we have learned, have many layers, and each needs to be properly addressed and balanced.

As for how much exercise or movement is right for us, there are many sources that offer various guidelines. Consult these as you see fit. I personally don't want to get into a numbers game with exercise, just like with nutrition. You need to move, period. What often scares people off from regular exercise are the rigid guidelines that dictate a certain amount of aerobic exercise so many times a week, and another amount of resistance training so many times a week, etc. Like all guidelines, these can be helpful, but despite the fact that we want details when it comes to everything based on our reductionist mindset, those details all too often end up working against us in the end. For the sake of a reference point, a thirty-minute, brisk walk or similar moderate activity should be the minimum you aim for each day. The reality, as often mentioned in these pages, is that we are dynamic, and we lead dynamic lives. One week, you may be able to do five days of one-hour aerobic classes but only one in another week. One month, you may sign up for a thirty-day yoga challenge, doing one-hour yoga classes daily, but in another month, you may barely get a weekly yoga class in. Whether it is aerobic, flexibility, or strength training—the three most fundamental types of physical movement—I repeat my point: You need to move, period. Make a serious effort to engage in meaningful movement daily, and regularly choose between activities that naturally engage each of the types of physical exercises to work all parts of your body accordingly.

Sleep

The right quality and quantity of sleep is needed each day for optimal health and prevention. When our bodies are out of balance and our health is already suffering in some way, we must pay even more special attention to our sleeping habits. Statistics show that too many of us are not getting enough sleep, and this heavily contributes to our health and weight problems. According to a 2013 Gallup poll, while 59 percent of U.S. adults meet the recommended amount of sleep, in 1942, 84 percent of the population did.[5] As our lifestyles took on more complexity and noise and became more mentally draining, it became more important than ever to sleep adequately. Yet, the opposite occurred; we are sleeping less today than we used to, with at least a third of us not getting enough deep, healthy sleep. We also have to factor in that while many report getting the standard recommended amount, this may not be enough for them. The Centers for Disease Control and Prevention state that insufficient sleep is a public health epidemic and that, aside from increased risk of various accidents, people suffering from insufficient sleep are more likely to suffer from chronic diseases such as hypertension, diabetes, depression, obesity, cancer, increased mortality, and reduced quality of life and productivity.[6]

The reasons for our insufficient or poor quality sleep are many. Some of us try our best but either cannot fall asleep, stay asleep continuously, or sleep long enough, usually due to some stress, worry, or anxiety. Some of us have various physical and chemical factors working against our ability to sleep properly, like side effects of pharmaceuticals, hormonal imbalances, excess weight, unhealthy sleep environments, etc. All too many of us try to stretch the hours of each day, decreasing the amount of time dedicated to sleep.

Common guidelines suggest that between seven to nine hours, on average eight hours, of sleep are necessary for good health on a physical, mental, and emotional level. It may be a great guideline but still leaves many of us today waking up feeling tired. This is why, as always, our primary guideline should be listening to our body and adjusting accordingly to our lifestyle needs. For example, those of us who do highly cognitive work would benefit from more sleep, as would those who are dealing with some major stress, trauma, or illness. If you wake up feeling tired, groggy, or irritable, chances are that you need more sleep. According to the National Sleep Foundation, there is no magic number when it comes to the right amount of sleep.[7] Researchers are learning that two factors govern our individual sleep need: *basal sleep need*—the amount of sleep our bodies need on a regular basis for optimal performance—and *sleep debt*— the accumulated sleep that is lost due to various causes. A basal sleep amount of eight hours is common for most of us, but the extra sleep necessary on top of that will be unique, based on our individual sleep debt. Many of us would benefit from two or more hours on top of our basal sleep need to properly recover and restore our body.

When it comes to sleep, its quality must be factored in as well. You may get nine hours of sleep, but if that sleep is disturbed, where you repeatedly wake-up, toss and turn, it may not be as effective as seven hours of good, solid sleep. Sleep is composed of several distinct non-REM (NREM) and REM stages, which we cycle through about four or five times each night. These stages play important roles in our restoration.

The hour when you fall asleep makes a big difference as well. First, it is optimal to respect our natural circadian rhythm. Obviously this poses a big challenge for those who have to work during the night in unnatural shifts. Melatonin, commonly known as the sleep hormone, which regulates our circadian rhythm, is naturally released around dusk. Within about an hour or two, we get naturally drowsy, and this is the ideal time to go to sleep. If we push through this timeframe, it is common to experience difficulty falling asleep. Sitting in front of a bright, electronic device into the night hours can further interfere with our sleep process. Generally speaking, the ideal time to go to sleep is definitely before midnight, around ten p.m. or earlier. The reasons for this go beyond an easier ability to fall asleep. The ten p.m.-to-two a.m. window is considered the most valuable, for it is when your immune system and key repair hormones do their jobs to physically repair the body and recharge organs like the adrenals, liver, and gallbladder. This is also the time when your melatonin hormone is at its highest concentration, and this influences a cascade of benefits. As renowned author and medical doctor, Christiane Northrup explains: sleep is one of the most effective ways to combat stress and high adrenaline levels. Adrenal fatigue, or burnout, is a serious issue for many adults today, especially women, and it can lead to weight gain and all sorts of health problems. Our adrenals typically recharge during the eleven p.m. to one a.m. timeframe.

There is no doubt that sleep is highly healing and restorative. It allows your body the time it needs to do most of its repair work, thereby making it one of the best methods for healing and prevention. When we regularly limit this, it has profound consequences on our entire state of health. Sleep also offers a highly effective detoxification for our body, thanks to its natural period of fasting. This is one of the reasons why it is common to experience a bowel movement first thing in the morning, as the body tries to eliminate and clean out what it processed overnight. To best support this natural fast and detoxification, it is optimal to leave about twelve hours between our last meal of the day and first meal of the next morning. This gives your body an uninterrupted time to properly work, heal, and repair. Recall that digestion is a taxing process, which takes away from the body's many balancing and healing processes. It is one of the main reasons why we lose our appetite when we are ill, and many holistic therapies, going back to the ancient times of Hippocrates, recommend minimal, light, mostly liquid nourishment, if not outright fasting, during periods of illness. As mentioned, sleep provides a time for your organs and brain to reset; this is why we wake up from healthy sleep feeling refreshed and rejuvenated. Like digestion, thinking, particularly analytical or incessant, is taxing on the body and mind. As we will cover in the meditation and mindfulness sections later in this chapter, one of the reasons why meditation is so healing and beneficial is that it can provide a rejuvenating rest for the mind, something most of us need today more so than ever.

As with exercise, some research warns about having too much of a good thing when it comes to sleep. Although this is highly debatable and not a concern for most of us. There are times when sleeping between ten to twelve hours may be required by our bodies for deep healing and restoration. If you regularly find yourself sleeping prolonged periods and/or still wake up feeling tired, though, it would be a good idea to consult with your healthcare provider, as this can be indicative of health problems. Finally, for those of us who enjoy or are able to take a nap, feel free to do so. Whether fifteen or forty-five minutes, we can benefit from an increased state of alertness and feeling refreshed. Naps can be especially valuable for parents of young children, who are not able to get a full night's rest. The most important thing is to listen to your body and respect its needs. The right quality and quantity of sleep is vital for optimal health, and we must make it a priority in our lives. An optimally healthy diet and quality of sleep go hand in hand. The better the quality of our food, the better the body we build to regulate and heal itself optimally, and the less toxins and nutritional stress we give it to have to deal with in the first place. This results in better sleep, better energy levels, and overall wellbeing.

Personal Care

What you put on your body should be taken just as seriously as what you put into it. There are tens of thousands of synthetic chemicals circulating amongst all the products today, including the personal care products we put onto our body daily. As I shared with you in Chapter 1, toxicity is one of the leading causes for many internal imbalances. Numerous personal care ingredients have been linked to various cancers, allergies, immune system suppression, skin disorders, hormonal imbalances, thyroid imbalances, and even infertility. What we often forget, or perhaps neglect to consider, is that our skin is a living, breathing organ, and most of what you put on your body gets into your body. This is far from an externally isolated issue, where perhaps some kind of skin irritation would be our biggest problem. This is a whole-body problem that impacts our health and weight in ways I feel we are just starting to fully recognize. We also know that our obsession with trying to keep ourselves clean is often a leading contributor to many imbalances in our natural microflora communities, never mind over-drying for the skin, which then necessitates the use of more products. Beneficial bacteria, for example, whether on our skin or in our intestines, designed to keep us healthy and balanced, are being destroyed by our many synthetic ingredients, leaving us vulnerable to various problems.

It is so important to make personal care part of our optimally healthy lifestyle habits to support healing and prevention in our synthetic, modern world. The best part is that we have plenty of choices. There are many natural and green personal care product companies that offer a wide assortment of products. Due to their increased popularity, prices have also become much more comparable to conventional synthetic products. Even though some green products are still pricier, the cost is usually easy to justify when we minimize how many products we use and their subsequent amounts, which brings us to a very important point.

The number-one rule of optimally healthy personal care is to minimize: reduce how many products you use and how much of each. While soap, shampoo, and toothpaste are pretty standard necessities, perfumes, body washes, hairstyling products, and mouthwash are not. Antiperspirants, for example, are some of the most problematic personal care products, and this is not only because of their harmful ingredients. The fact is that they directly and intentionally impede one of your body's main and best detoxification systems. As described by the research and experiments of Bruce Lourie and Rick Smith in their book, *Toxin Toxout*, perspiration is often more effective at eliminating toxic chemicals from our bodies than urination. You may gasp with panic at the thought of going without an antiperspirant, but you might find it interesting that body odor is usually very reflective of the body's internal state of toxicity or imbalance. This applies to our oral health and odor as well. The more you clean out and support your body with wholesome plant foods, natural personal care products, and healthy lifestyles, the more you will notice a difference in the quality of your perspiration and health. Natural deodorants are plenty today, and while they will not stop you from sweating (actually a good thing), they will mask odors with varying success. Ultimately, we can try to eliminate or mask our odors with the latest and greatest mouthwash or antiperspirant, but these do not address the underlying health imbalances, they only compound them further.

Back to our personal care in general, even for those of us in the population who choose to wear cosmetics, we have an abundance of natural companies and options to choose from in this area as well. We do not need to inhale or absorb more toxins, and in the case of lipsticks, balms, and glosses, actually ingest more compounds that will work against our health. Simplify, minimize, and free yourself from tedious personal care routines. Connect more mindfully with your body, with how it looks naturally, how it functions, and learn to love your body as it is, without feeling the need to mask it with all sorts of things. The more you support your body on both an internal and external level, the more your body will show it, in the quality of your skin, hair, nails, or even how gracefully you age. When people compliment you on your glowing skin, it won't be because of some overpriced cream with questionable effects; rather, it will be the result of you supporting your body as it was meant to be supported, from the inside out.

The second rule of thumb to optimize this area, once you have simplified your personal care routine, is to choose products that are the most natural and the least harmful. As mentioned, many green personal care companies exist today. Of course, as with any other popular market, exploitation is common. Even many popular personal care brand name giants, who have been making chemical personal care for decades, try to lure us in with words like "natural," "herbal," or even "organic," but don't be fooled. One look at the ingredient list, and you can easily tell it is all part of a clever marketing scheme to make a product look and sound better. This can all seem quite overwhelming, as the onus is on you to be a knowledgeable and responsible consumer, but there are several things you can do. Visit your local natural health food store and familiarize yourself with some of the brands they carry. Talk to the sales staff and see what feedback they've received and what they recommend as real and worthy green options. You can also do a quick search online for the top-ten most toxic ingredients to avoid in your personal care products. I have created several resources on my site www.evolvingwellness.com to help you navigate this area, and ewg.org has one of the best freely accessible databases about the toxicity of specific products and/or ingredients. Finally, seek out local artisans in your area who are making high-quality, natural personal care products. Soaps, lip or body balms, scrubs, and various moisturizers are some of the easiest products to make. They are increasingly being made at home by health-conscious consumers, who then turn their personal endeavors into small businesses that we can support, while supporting our health.

Your Relationships

Aside from our personal lifestyle choices, relationships have a huge impact on our health and the state of healing or prevention. They are often our greatest source of stress, so they can be very destructive to our overall health and wellbeing. Just like there are toxic ingredients in food or personal care, there are toxic relationships. By taking the journey into optimal health, you are taking steps toward honoring and respecting your mind, body, *and* spirit. Do an honest inventory of your relationships. Are you still immersed in a friendship that has run its course, where both of you have gone in different directions but are still trying to force things to work simply out of some unspoken or assumed obligation? Is a romantic partnership weighing you down and limiting your state of being, as opposed to uplifting you to express your highest potential? Is there a family member with an unhealthy dependency or who fails to respect your personal boundaries? Are you someone that people have a hard time getting along with, someone who creates constant drama for others? All of these are important questions to consider during some of our regular and very necessary contemplation times.

The first thing we need to understand when it comes to our relationships is that they can be a valuable platform for our personal growth and evolution. The answer is never to simply run away when a relationship challenge presents itself; rather, try to work with it and understand its role. Yes, life is full of challenges, and we don't have a say about many of them, but we always have a say about how we respond to anything that comes our way. The first place to start to improve this area and your quality of life is with mindfulness. We will talk more about this later in this chapter and in Chapter 20. Every day, regardless of who you are with, you can consciously choose to act from a place of love, compassion, kindness, and understanding or from one of anger, hostility, ignorance, and irritation. If you are having a hard time expressing your truth, your feelings, or your needs, you need to pay attention to that and work to strike a happy balance for yourself; emotional suppression has many ties to all sorts of diseases and ills. If you are over-expressive or impulsive, often failing to consider the consequences of your words or actions, the same thing applies.

The most important place to start for successful, joyous, and peaceful relationships is with yourself. There is ample literature today about how negative thoughts and perceptions of ourselves can be very destructive forces in our lives. If you do not honor, respect, value, and love yourself, this will be accordingly reflected in your diet, relationships, work, and other areas of your life. We know we have a serious problem with selfishness in our society, as the state of our humanity, environment, and planet greatly reflects this. Perhaps partly due to this and perhaps due to other conditioning, we are not taught healthy self-love while growing up. This is detrimental to our wellbeing, and it is one of the reasons why we seek love and pleasure from the external so much, be it from our food or the people in our lives. It is ironic, in a sense, that in order to be more selfless, inclusive, caring, compassionate, and empathic, we need to start with self-love. As the saying goes, you cannot give to another what you do not have or cannot give to yourself. I will share an example from above to illustrate this point further: Trying to become a better person by focusing externally before focusing internally is like trying to create better skin using external products rather than internal building blocks. Everything starts from the inside and radiates out. Many of us think it is easier to love others than it is to love ourselves, but this is not quite as it appears. Such love is very conditional, limited, and possessive; thus, it is the cause of many problems and friction in our lives. It is most often filled with expectations, and when these are not met in the way we envisioned, this spearheads all sorts of feelings of animosity. When we learn to become whole ourselves, the source of our own love and joy, life takes on a completely different meaning. We will think, speak, and act differently. We will also interact differently, not just with other people, but with all beings on this planet, all of nature. We will make different choices that are naturally more in alignment with our being, our bodies, and our planet. We will not be easily influenced or confused by external sources and their various hypes, claims, or promises. We will have a better sense of who we are and what we need, and we will take appropriate steps to make that happen. This is why one of my biggest pieces of advice, above and beyond any healthy eating advice, is to take the journey of self-love seriously; when this becomes your guiding factor, everything else will naturally and almost effortlessly begin to fall into place.

Your Work

Most of us have something in our daily life that we call work. Whether you are running your own business, working for someone else, or a homemaker, your work is important. Nevertheless, you cannot allow your work to become your life or run it. It is just one of the things you do in how you choose to express yourself on this planet. Whenever we attach our identity too strongly to a thing, person, or event, we set ourselves up for great suffering. This doesn't mean we shouldn't fully engage in our work or enjoy it; rather, the essence of our being and what creates true joy and fulfillment must always will come from within. If you find yourself consumed by your work, it is a good time for some deep, reflective life assessment. Next to relationships, our work can be one of the greatest sources of our stress, so it is another key area that needs to be consciously addressed by us. Each day, people in our society choose to revolve their life around their work, putting aside their health, relationships, and balance, only to one day be given some news or a diagnosis that stops them in their tracks. We don't have to wait to find ourselves in such a situation to make some meaningful changes. Redefine what success and happiness mean to you. Reprioritize your life today, right now, while you are most empowered to do so. Don't wait like far too many do, only to live with regret and remorse.

Second, when it comes to your work, it is a well-known fact that the level of creativity, meaning, and satisfaction that we live with daily has a big impact on the state of our health. If your work doesn't feel joyous, if you don't feel like you are adding value or that your work has much meaning, or if you don't have enough creative balance in your life, reassess your choices. Many of us get stuck in places or positions that stopped being rewarding or fulfilling a long time ago, but we fail to move on, fearing a loss of comfort and security. Life is based on ever-evolving change. Know that there are always choices—always—and the first step to finding out what amazing potential or experiences await you is to have enough courage to discover and consider those choices. One of the easiest ways to feel confident or comfortable enough to follow through on other choices often involves the restructuring of our lifestyle, namely in the way of simplification. Each day, an increasing number of people on this planet, myself included, make the choice to simplify our lives and minimize the external obligations that rob us of our personal freedom. Let's face it: The bigger the square footage of your home, debt, or responsibilities related to your material possessions, the more resources are needed to upkeep them. When we say we have no choice and claim we have to stay in a certain life-draining job, we are actually making a choice, the choice *not* to change. Perhaps we are afraid or are just reluctant to make choices that will provide us with more creativity, joy, or freedom, normally because we have attached our identity to a certain way of life. However, if we reexamine that way of life and our priorities, the next steps to take seem to be self-explanatory. Ultimately, don't let your work destroy your health or life. It really, really isn't worth it. If you feel or know a shift is needed in this area, connect with people and resources, whether a good friend or an inspirational book, that will support you and offer help on your quest to make the changes you seek.

Nature

One of the most healing environments on this planet is nature. It doesn't matter if it is an ocean shore lined with palm trees, a mountain ridge lined with conifers, an open field of wild grasses, a local park with some trees and flowers, or your back yard composed of a lawn and shrubs. Where there are natural components like grasses, trees, flowers, and animals, where there is contact with Earth, an emphasis on the air, sun, and sky, and especially where there is a higher concentration of natural-to-manmade components, there is restorative and therapeutic value. Studies can prove the numerous benefits of nature on our health, but most of us already know this firsthand. We may not be able to explain it, but we just feel better and more relaxed when we are outdoors, in natural spaces. One of the most notable, extensive books on this topic is *Your Brain on Nature*, by medical Dr. Eva M. Selhub and naturopathic Dr. Alan C. Logan. In the book, the doctors examine the scientific discoveries related to the way in which nature immersion and deprivation impacts our health and wellbeing, including the ways in which our disconnection from nature, driven in part by screen-based gadgetry technology, may be shaping our attitudes as a society about nature. When it comes to our cognitive function alone, there is a big reason why nature elicits a calming, healing, and less stressful reaction on our overall wellbeing: Nature grabs our attention in an effortless, modest, bottom-up fashion, allowing top-down, directed-attention abilities a chance to recharge. Manmade environments, on the other hand, grab our attention in a forced, dramatic way and additionally require directed attention, making them more draining and less restorative. A 2008 study published in *Psychological Science* reported that time spent in nature or even looking at pictures of nature can improve directed-attention abilities, improving our concentration and validating the *attention restoration theory*.[8] From lower blood pressure to lower stress responses, from increased calmness to increased creativity, the associated benefits of nature are many. We also have information about the many positive health and healing effects from having actual physical, bare skin contact with Earth. The documentary *Grounded* and its sequel offer excellent resources on this topic. Whether your body is immersed in a body of water or your bare feet are touching Earth, there is actual research showing how and why this benefits our wellbeing. Again, our ancestors knew this naturally, but most of us need to relearn what should be innate to us. This information comes at a crucial time, as our society is inundated with many stressors and components that cause all sorts of physical, mental, emotional, and energetic imbalance and damage. Take the different risks associated with electromagnetic fields (EMF) and our various technology devices alone. For those of us who spend most of our time indoors, on electronic devices, amongst high concentrations of many electromagnetic waves, it has, perhaps, never been more important than now to set aside time for regular trips outdoors, specifically time for thorough grounding.

Whether you passively sit and relax in nature, or actively engage in some activity, you can still enjoy the many benefits it offers for healing, prevention, and optimal wellbeing. While most of us don't need convincing on this subject and would readily spend more time in nature if our schedules allowed, a small subset of the population does not feel the same. There are those of us who are uncomfortable, so to speak, with nature's various elements. There may also be a lot of fear associated with nature, and this is often the underlying foundation of this discomfort. Fear of touching the wrong plant, being stung by an insect, coming across a wild animal, fear of the elements, and fear of natural dirt are all common. Most of these fears are completely unfounded and stem from our disconnected way of life. We sterilize our homes, try to sterilize our lives, and want to exhibit a sense of control over anything in our reach. Nature, however, does not work this way. She may seem unpredictable and even dangerous, but that is only until we get to know her. To her, everything comes down to balance and maintaining harmony for all. A certain level of reverence and respect is essential when interacting with her, and this seems to be a missing component for too many of us. We need to understand that we are not above nature; we are simply one small part of her, neither more or less important than any of the others. Another thing we have not yet learned or have forgotten is that it is a futile task to try to control nature. We can see this clearly on many fronts, and it only comes back to harm us. Our attempts with pesticides (various insecticides, herbicides, etc.) and genetic modification aimed at trying to control some elements of nature, are a prime example. We have destroyed and continue to destroy ecosystems, polluting our air, water, and ourselves. All the while, the so-called pests simply find ways to adapt, forcing us to implement stronger and usually more destructive measures. To a large degree, the idea of pests is rooted in unhealthy farming practices, like monocultures and depleted soils. Still we don't seem to get it: The answer is not in fighting against nature but in working with it to arrive at favorable outcomes for all.

Whatever your relationship is with nature at this time, there is no doubt in my mind that optimal health necessitates the element of nature. If your busy schedule holds you back from spending more quality time in nature, I invite you to reprioritize your choices. We can choose a tiring walk in a shopping mall, bombarded by artificial sights, sounds, and smells, or we can choose a revitalizing walk in nature, stimulated by natural sights, sounds, and smells.

If it is any kind of fear that is holding you back from spending more quality time in nature, educate yourself on the topic at hand. Wild animal attacks, for example, are often sensationalized by our media, as if animals are all vicious predators, hoping to attack us, while nothing could be further from the truth. Threatening wild animal encounters are rare, for starters, and if given a choice, nearly every animal prefers to take flight rather than fight. The intelligence of other beings is just now being more fully investigated, and the results show astonishing results so far. A 2014 study by researchers from Oxford University has shown that even fruit flies exhibit a thinking-before-acting behavior, especially for more complex decision-making, rather than acting solely on instinct.[9] Imagine what that means for more complex organisms. Their levels of mental and emotional processing are yet to be fully understood and appreciated by us. Their relationships with us often go astray, too, due to our treatment of them and their habitats, as well as a general lack of respect and understanding about their needs and behaviors. If we are to thrive on Planet Earth into the future decades and centuries to come, it will take a serious paradigm shift when it comes to our relationship with and our treatment of nature.

As we touched upon in Chapter 16 when discussing Vitamin D, the sun is essential for our health, being correlated with healing and prevention rather than disease creation. If this is a common fear or concern for you, learn more about this topic and the sun's vital role in your health. Practice sun-smart habits to thrive, which include covering up with light clothing or using natural sunblock options when needed. We know the air quality in nature is better than what our synthetic chemical-filled homes or congested city centers can offer. We know real, pure, natural springs are still able to offer us the best drinking water possible, something no filtered water can compete with. We know the beauty and harmony of nature directly speaks to our souls and invigorates us on a mind-body-spirit level. Hence, make regular time in nature, whether for a few minutes each day or a few successive hours each week. This must be part of your optimally healthy lifestyle. You don't need to be limited by financial resources, as your back yard or local park can even offer benefits. We don't need to be limited by the seasons, either, as nature offers gifts in every season. As long as we approach her consciously, respecting the natural elements and our bodies' specific needs, we can safely enjoy the richness, serenity, and opportunity she offers.

Meditation

In our busy, noisy worlds, where we are inundated by all sorts of stimuli, conscious time-outs are essential for optimal health and wellbeing. For the purpose of our discussion, we'll refer to these as "meditation," but if you are not comfortable with that term for any reason, you can simply refer to this practice as stillness, reflection, or contemplation time. It is not mere coincidence that there has been such a rise in popularity of yoga over the past several decades. While our Western world sees it mainly as a physical activity, the entire foundation of yoga is based on meditation and a conscious approach to life, which meditation facilitates. One of the main roles of the physical activity is to prepare the body for meditation. Whether yoga, actual meditation, or similar practices, we continue to see a rise in all these areas, as many are recognizing that we have tapped ourselves out energetically and spiritually. We are running on empty, and it shows. Eastern cultures and traditions have, for millennia, honored and prioritized the inward path, seeking balance between the inner and outer worlds. Our Western approach has been exceedingly outward. We base our entire lives on external sources of meaning and pleasure, such as material possessions, fame, money, people, and food. If for no other reason than our personal health and happiness, we need to reevaluate our approach.

Making time for silence and stillness in your life will go a long way. Whether you want to practice some kind of formal meditation or not, we can all use some focused quiet time. You can start with a daily habit of taking ten to fifteen minutes for yourself, perhaps at the very start or very end of your day. You can be indoors or in nature. You can be in complete silence or in the presence of gentle, non-vocal music. You can sit on the floor or on a chair. It is preferable to keep the spine straight, but not to lie down, lest you fall asleep. While sleep is not a bad thing and offers the benefits we discussed earlier, it does not offer the same benefits that we can specifically get from meditation or focused, contemplative time. You can observe your thoughts and/or breath, you can choose to reflect on something, or you can contemplate something of importance to you. Aside from what ancient peoples already knew, modern science now backs up the many positive benefits of various types of meditation on our brain function, overall health, healing, and wellbeing. One of the pioneers of scientific research on meditation is Jon Kabat-Zinn PhD, Founding Executive Director of the Center for Mindfulness in Medicine, Healthcare, and Society. His research has shown numerous health benefits linked specifically to mindfulness meditation. Some types of meditation exercises appear to have calming effects on the sympathetic nervous system, the fight-or-flight response, while activating the parasympathetic nervous system relaxation response.[10] Meditation can help to decrease anxiety, worry, and rumination, thus helping us to sleep better. It can empower us on our journey of self-love, optimal health, creativity, healing, and many other areas. One of the key reasons, though, why I most recommend meditation is for its ability to foster mindfulness. The higher our state of mindful awareness, the easier, more coherent, and harmonious our lives become, which brings us to the next section.

Mindfulness

I really cannot stress enough the importance of mindfulness, which is why it is mentioned more than once in this book. In its simplest usage, this means exactly what it sounds like: operating from a state that uses the mind. You may think you always use your mind when you think, speak, and make decisions, but this is not as simple as it seems. It depends what part of the mind we use and to what degree. As we will cover in Chapter 20, the part of the mind you use—conscious versus subconscious—makes all the difference here, but there are other elements to consider as well. More formally, mindfulness is defined as the practice of intentional, nonjudgmental awareness of moment-to-moment experiences. In other words, seeing things as they truly are, not how we think they should or could be, and being unattached to the outcome. Mindfulness can also be understood as a state of heightened awareness or consciousness. Those of you who are already familiar with this concept and have made the development of this quality and state of being a focused part of your life can relate to why it is life transforming.

The practice of mindfulness is commonly employed as a therapy for various mental and emotional imbalances within the field of psychology. Other science and research areas that are exploring its connection to our health, stress reduction, and wellbeing are arriving at the same conclusions when it comes to the many benefits of mindfulness. As I've mentioned before, if there is one sure way to drastically improve the quality of your life, and, thus health, it is by becoming more mindful.

You begin to live with an increasingly positive amount of conscious thoughts, words, and actions and a decreasing amount of regret, guilt, and shame. You take responsibility for your choices and have an easier time seeing the consequences of any action, thereby taking the actions that lead to the most desired consequences for you. With respect to food, you don't get caught up in impulsive, emotional, or unconscious eating. You are fully aware of what you eat, how much, and why. As you can imagine, this will do wonders for your weight and your entire state of health. With an increased state of mindfulness, you are empowered to consciously create your life and improve your responses to the surprises that life often offers. You are no longer engulfed in victimhood or blaming your external surroundings; rather, you take an active role in the creation of your life. You become more resilient and courageous, for you begin to understand that regardless of what happens, you always have the choice of how to perceive it and act in response to it. You are no longer a slave to your thoughts and emotions. You have an easier time catching destructive thoughts and guiding your mind back to seek constructive states of being. As we will discuss in the next chapter, all of this has a tremendous benefit for your physical, mental, and emotional health.

But how does one become mindful? The best part of mindfulness is that, while many tools and techniques exist to develop this skill, it can be instantaneously experienced by each of us. Take this moment, for example. As you are reading, become aware of your body, how it feels right now, where it is positioned, any sounds or scents around you, and just observe with awareness. This is the underlying nature of mindfulness: being present to what is. We can invoke it anytime we choose. The trick is really just to be mindful enough to switch into a mindful state of being and not be consumed by unconscious or habitual mind patterns that often fixate us on the past or future. This is where those tools and techniques can come in handy to help you cultivate a regular mindfulness practice. *Mindfulness meditation* is one of the primary techniques to train this quality within us. Other techniques include yoga, tai chi, and qigong. In a sense, it can be considered mind training; our minds require training because they generally operate in an uncontrolled, chaotic fashion. The mind is our tool, yet left unchecked it thinks what it wants to think, normally based on faulty conditioning, sparking all sorts of emotional reactions, some pleasant and others not so much. Think about it (pun intended): Would you consciously choose to think negative thoughts about yourself? Would you consciously choose to think negatively about another human being? Would you consciously choose to worry? For most of us, the answers are a definite no. In fact, that is one of the things I often hear from people when I address the futile nature of worrying, that they cannot help it, but therein lies our main point! We carry the idea that so many of our thoughts and emotions are immanent, that they cannot be changed or stopped, and, worse yet, that they are presumably natural. There is nothing natural about a mind that is running your life and destroying the quality of your life. We've collectively accepted this as a norm in our distracted society, but we are now coming to the realization that there is another way. We need to be in charge of our minds, not let them be in charge of us.

While mindfulness is often deeply desired by those who understand its potential, many of us are not willing to put the necessary effort required to attain it. Again, knowing something and actually applying it are two very different things. Like with any other new skill, it takes practice. With regular repetition and practice, you can continuously grow and sharpen this ability, until it becomes a part of your life, second nature to you. It doesn't stop there though. Life is amazing in its design, in that it always offers us more room for growth, to practice this skill and continue to refine it, reaching ever-higher levels of mindfulness. As with self-love, most of us are not taught this as children growing up in today's world. In fact, our society pretty much depends on you not being mindful. After all, a mindful person can easily see through the games, propaganda, and illusions. There is so much more that can be said on this topic, however, this is not a book on mindfulness but optimal nutrition. I therefore encourage you to explore this topic in more detail via other sources, as may be pertinent to you. You can start by visiting mindful.org, an initiative that shares information and resources for being mindful in all aspects of daily living. Through our discussion here, my intention was simply to bring this to your awareness, to alert you to its necessary inclusion as part of optimally healthy lifestyle habits.

For many of us, depending on our backgrounds, this topic may feel ambiguous. Not to worry, for every journey has its time, and all you need to do right now is focus on what resonates most with you. In this book, and in this chapter alone, I have provided you with many guidelines for optimally healthy eating and living. Choose and act on what you are most ready for. You may wish to tackle it all, and that would be wonderful, but be sure not to get overwhelmed in trying to do too much too fast. Take the steps that feel most in tune with you, and make your journey an enjoyable one. We have enough challenges in our lives; healthy eating and living should be a welcome addition, not another source of stress. How we go about it will ultimately depend on our choice of perceptions and conscious thoughts, words, and actions.

CHAPTER 20
The Mind-Body Connection

On our journey into optimal health, weight, and wellness, we have come to the last chapter, and there is a purposeful reason for this information being placed at the end. When I actively began my personal and professional journey into the field of nutrition, I was awed by how powerful our food can be at healing us, preventing disease, and helping us maintain optimal health. I wanted to shout it from the rooftops, and I couldn't understand why it was not already the societal prime focus for keeping us healthy and well. Sadly, I quickly learned about how our system, our governments, industry, and regulating bodies work when it comes to handling food, nutrition, and health. Basically put, we've allowed corporations to run our society, and we are paying a hefty price for it.

I used to think governments had the power to enforce better rules or laws when it came to food and nutrition. I was dismayed to find that they often choose to please and appease corporate interests over public welfare. As the years went on, I learned that, more often than not, their hands are tied, even if they do actually want to implement some positive policies, with consumer health as the main priority. This was one of the guiding reasons why I became so passionate about educating people about their food and health; I realized that in the end, it all comes down to personal responsibility. Our food, nutrition, and health system may be far from effective, never mind perfect, but no one is forcing us to eat, drink, or address our health in a destructive way. At the end of the day, we still have choices, but in order to exercise them, we must become informed, conscious, and discerning consumers.

During my period of nutritional enlightenment, as I'll call it, equipped with the knowledge about the immense healing and preventative power of food, I wanted to believe that if applied correctly, we could all enjoy optimal health, weight, and wellbeing. However, as the years went on, another big revelation began to unravel. Piece by piece, from both personal and professional experience, I learned that, as important as our diet is, there is something above and beyond it that is even more powerful: our mind. To summarize this in the simplest way possible, there is no diet perfect enough to compete with a mind (state of being) that is rooted in negativity, fear, anger, jealousy, resentment, despair, hopelessness, exhaustion, or similar destructive states.

When our bodies manifest or express a disease, it is after a state of imbalance has existed within for some time (days, weeks, months, or years). Usually, albeit not necessarily, the more destructive the disease, the longer the state of imbalance has been in effect. We can create an imbalance in our body, moving it away from its natural state of balance (homeostasis) and good health through our food and drink choices, exposure to toxins, lack of sleep, and unhealthy lifestyle habits. However, at the root of any and every disease or imbalance manifestation, there is a mind component that works via our thoughts, beliefs, perceptions, emotions, and feelings. As author and mind-body expert Lise Bourbeau shares in her book, *Your Body's Telling You: Love Yourself!*:

"When illness or dis-ease is indicated, the body is communicating to us that our way of thinking (although unconscious) is out of harmony with what is beneficial to our being. Illness indicates the need for change in our belief system and tells us that we have reached our physical and psychological limits."

In this chapter, we will briefly explore the mind-body connection. If you are already familiar with how it works, my hope is that this section will trigger you to work consciously and actively with your mind to attain full-spectrum optimal health and wellbeing. If you are new to this idea, I recommend looking into the work of other experts who have dedicated entire books and/or their life's work to this field, like Lise Bourbeau or Drs. Christiane Northrup, Elaine R. Ferguson, and Bernie Siegel, as well as many quantum science and metaphysical experts.

Before we explore the mind-body connection, though, there are two other areas that need our attention to understand the mind's role in our ability to make smart, healthy choices when it comes to our food, and life in general.

Infectious Mind Patterns

In order to help you gain a further understanding of the nature of the mind and how it can work for or against us, we will begin by examining the infectious nature of ideas and transfer of information within cultures. This body of work is called *memetics*. Our purpose in this discussion is not to examine or dissect this field; rather, we will rely on its basic premise to better understand our personal way of thinking about food and health.

In *Virus of the Mind*, Richard Brodie describes how ideas are created and transferred to become cultural paradigms, true or not. He calls these "viruses of the mind" and explains that understanding memetics can help us better understand ourselves, how our society works, and how to avoid being manipulated or taken advantage of. This is especially vital for our discussion when it comes to the marketing and messages produced by the food and beverage industry, corporations, and many so-called health-based experts. The first step in empowering ourselves comes from understanding that many of our current ideas, if not most of them, are simply not our own. We adopt them, becoming infected with the ideas of others and subconsciously make them our own. When this has a positive effect on our lives, there is no harm done. However, when this has a negative effect on us, it works to our disadvantage.

The biggest problem with unconsciously accepting information or being conditioned into a certain way of thinking is that it forms beliefs that may not be true at all, beliefs that will begin to govern our lives in deleterious ways. This impacts our choices and alters our behavior in ways that can work against us and others, to varying degrees. It can create confusion, contradiction, and controversy, as well as animosity amongst those who derive their sense of identity from these ideas. One glance at any popular website's comments section on almost any topic drives this point home. When we believe something strongly enough, it begins to form the basis of our reality. Regardless of what anyone else may say, we consider it part of our foundational understanding, and we may feel threatened or insulted or defensive when we sense that someone else is challenging what we consider to be truth. The interesting thing about this is that when it really is our truth, in the sense that we fully understand what we think or believe and why, we are not likely to feel threatened by anyone else's difference of opinion or ideology. It is always valuable to consider all these aspects from both your and the other party's perspective, fostering a greater sense of empathy amongst our human race. To do this, though, we need our conscious mind rather than our conditioned one.

What memetics reveals is that viruses of the mind (thoughts and beliefs) do not grow or gain cultural acceptance based on truth rather based on the success of transmission and acceptance. As you can likely deduce, this has profound consequences on every area of our society. For our purposes, though, we will focus on how it impacts food and nutrition. Let's examine some common mind viruses as they pertain to our discussion. Protein being synonymous with meat or animal products is an excellent example of a mind virus. A multitude of people have been infected with the thought that not eating animal products equates with a lack of protein. Speaking of protein, in and of itself, this is another virus of the mind that has taken hold of many in various ways, some of which we covered in Chapter 17. Another great example comes from the book *Diet for a Small Planet*, written by Frances Moore Lappé in 1971. It implanted the idea of protein combining, which is still being rectified to this day. Similar problems exist for fat and carbohydrate mind viruses that have variably infected many. Whether it is the idea that dairy is the ideal for strong bones, that dessert follows a meal, or that gluten is public enemy number one, the examples are many. If we are going to accept or apply an idea, especially one that directly impacts the quality of our lives, we should properly look into it and examine both sides of the story. Unfortunately, most of us will not follow up in such a way, because it is easier to just accept an idea at face value, especially if it supports a habit that we wish to sustain or one that has some element of fear over us (i.e. missing out on the right nutrients).

Just looking back at my own life, I recall so many areas where I did a complete 180 with respect to the thoughts and beliefs I embodied. As children, we grow up learning our ideas and our beliefs from our parents, close family, and friends. At school, we begin to adopt the ideas taught to us by our teachers. Once we reach adulthood, especially in today's world of mass media and technology, most of the thoughts, beliefs, and paradigms we operate from are not our own. When I was working on my science degree, I inherently accepted most of the information I was being taught. I accepted that the food guide/pyramid provided the formula for healthy eating, that drugs were the answer to disease, and that our health was largely governed by external sources beyond our control. It wasn't until several years later that I began to consciously examine my thoughts and beliefs, that I experienced profound paradigm shifts. Some of these led me down the many avenues of holistic health, for which I will forever be grateful, as they transformed my life and how I understand health, nutrition, and, most importantly, my mind's and body's abilities. Today, whether it comes from the best expert, a book, or a study, I embrace nothing unless I have some supporting information about it. Most importantly, it must resonate with my inner knowing, and I recommend a similar approach to others for the purpose of empowerment, clarity, and discernment. We have become so detached from our inner guidance system that most of us do not even know what is best for us anymore. We need to come back to that inner sense of knowing. We need to find our truth, live it, and share it as we see fit. We may be inspired by the truth of another, but we should never blindly accept it as our own. Add it to your toolkit of supporting information, and work with it in ways that resonate with your inner being.

"Taking over bits of your mind and pulling you in different directions, mind viruses distract you from what's most important to you in life and cause confusion, stress, and even despair."

— Richard Brodie, *Virus of the Mind*

Every thought and belief can be challenged based on our unique experiences, perceptions, and biases. In the end, the answer is not to get everyone to agree, so don't hold your breath for every health and nutrition expert to subscribe to the same dietary prescription, although whole-food, plant-based comes close. The key is to find your own way, consciously, based on what makes most sense to you—not to your parents, your spouse, your community, or even your doctor. By all means, you should respect their input, just as they hopefully respect yours, but never lose your innate sense of knowing what is likely right and best for you. To expand your state of consciousness and strengthen your inner connection, it is vital to engage in mind-optimizing techniques, like meditation, yoga, tai chi, or qigong, as discussed in the previous chapter. These will help to train your mind to operate from a higher state of consciousness rather than conditioning. Have your mind work for you rather than against you.

The Quality of Your Mind

In the previous section, I shared with you about the importance of being a conscious, discerning thinker. This is effective advice, especially for today's times, but it is possible that despite our best intentions, we may not be able to access this ability to its fullest potential. The underlying cause of this is quite ironic. In order to make good food choices (or any good choices, for that matter), you need an optimally working brain. However, to have an optimally working brain, you need good food. There is no doubt in my mind that the better we eat, the better we think, and I am not alone in this observation. Although opinions vary as to what will create optimal brain function, many experts in this field concur that the quality of our nutrition is directly linked to our cognitive function, mental health, moods, and behavior.

Dr. Alan Logan has dedicated an entire book, *The Brain Diet*, to the scientific examination of the connection between diet and brain function. In it, he explains that two processes directly impede our brain function: oxidative stress and inflammation. You may recall from Chapter 1 that these are two of the main root causes of most of our physical imbalances and diseases. They are most directly linked to consuming too many refined sugars, refined grains, vegetable oils, and animal fat, while not getting enough phytonutrients, antioxidants, vitamins, and minerals from vegetables, fruits, whole grains, herbs, and spices. The guidance provided in this book fully supports these findings. Differences do exist on the topic of fish and fish oils, due to their controversial nature, as covered in Chapters 12 and 16. The common conclusion is to focus on whole, natural, plant foods that are rich in healthy macronutrients, micronutrients, phytonutrients, and antioxidants, as well as increasing the omega-3 food sources, while decreasing omega-6 food sources.

It is important to note that "brain" and "mind," while considered the same by many, are not being used interchangeably here. My personal research and experience is that they are two distinct entities that are intricately connected in ways that we have yet to fully understand. The brain is the physical and biochemical side; the mind is the psychological and emotional side. So, in the case of our nutrition, the quality of our food affects the quality of our brain function, and both affect the quality of our minds. Whichever way you choose to see it, there is ample supporting evidence today, aside from any personal experience you may have, which shows that the quality and quantity of our nutrition directly influences our cognitive abilities, memory, focus, clarity, and even our emotional wellbeing and moods. A 2008 article published in *Nature Reviews Neuroscience* reviewed over 160 research studies that examined these findings.[1] Speaking of emotional wellbeing, inadequate diets may impede our ability to effectively handle stress. For example, an increased risk of depression has been noted in those who eat refined carbohydrate and fast foods.[2]

Yes, we do keep returning to the same message, don't we? On a fundamental and practical level, this all makes sense. Your body, including all of its cells, tissues, organs, and biochemical substances is comprised of the food you consume. When we eat poor-quality, nutrient-deficient, chemically altered foods, they negatively impact our cognitive capacity. For many people in our society, this manifests as a regular state of brain fog, a feeling of confusion, forgetfulness, with lack of focus and mental clarity. It can also include irritability, hyperactivity, and mental fatigue, as well as a general lack of motivation, creativity, and ambition. As you can imagine, the unfortunate part is that this creates a vicious cycle. The worse we eat, the worse we think, and the worse we think, the worse our decision-making is, including when it comes to our food.

A diet that is natural, wholesome, and rich in valuable, nutrient-dense substances promotes optimal cognitive activity. Our way of thinking changes; we become more clear, coherent, and rational. Our decision-making and problem solving skills improve; we become more confident and resourceful. We find it easier to lead a more mindful, consciously driven life. We are better able to handle stress and emotional turmoil and face life's various challenges. We are more likely to adopt an optimistic mindset, and wake up with a sense of purpose, meaning, and drive. We naturally gravitate toward creativity and expressing ourselves in constructive, meaningful, positive ways. All of these aspects increase the quality of our lives, and should be a serious incentive to take what we put into our bodies that much more seriously.

The Manifestations of the Mind

While most of us agree that the mind has some influential effect on us and our lives, the power of the mind is still grossly underestimated amidst mainstream society. Leading-edge research and thinkers, however, are showing us more and more that the mind is at the root of our health and wellbeing. Recall our discussion on the meaning of healthy from Chapter 1, as well as that example everyone seems to have of the so-called perfectly healthy person who somehow succumbed to some serious disease. This is, in fact a perfect example not of what health or healthy mean but of the holistic nature of our state of being.

We are at the forefront of a major paradigm shift in our society when it comes to the nature of disease manifestation—really the manifestation of all things we consider our reality. If you look at conventional science and thinking alone, it appears to be business as usual in how we see and understand the manifestation, healing, or prevention of disease. However, when you begin to research what leading-edge thinkers, doctors, and scientists have discovered in just the last 100 years alone and continue to discover today, the story looks very different. Even though we are talking about health and nutrition, due to its holistic nature, which includes the mind, we find ourselves delving into the field of quantum physics. If this sounds intimidating, not to worry: My intention is to explain the basics in a way that can be easily understood to empower you and hopefully ignite a curiosity in you to explore these fields further. To begin to grasp the nature of the mind-body connection, we first have to understand what we (and all things, including thoughts) are made of, as well as the basics of our how our minds work and their connection to the body.

Our basic understanding begins at the physical level, as this is what we can most directly see and experience. Near the end of the seventeenth century, we learned that the cell is the basic unit of life of that we and all living things are made of; although the Buddha, Siddhārtha Gautama, seemed to know this thousands of years earlier. As our scientific technology advanced, we learned that cells are made up of various organelles that are comprised of various biochemicals: compounds and elements. Each element is made up of atoms, made up of protons, neutrons, and electrons, and each of these seem to be made up of yet smaller units. Our science today continues to probe these frontiers ever more deeply, as the journey inward and outward appears to be infinite, something most spiritual traditions already know. Either way, the nature of the atom is energy, so when we consider what we are made of, beyond organs, tissues, and cells, it is energy. But it doesn't stop there. Quantum science tells us that all physical reality is comprised of energy, including our thoughts and emotions! Everything has its own unique vibration, with a creative force of some sort, whether constructive or destructive. Therefore, our thoughts and emotions have an impact not only on our bodies but also on our surrounding environment and collective consciousness.

The power of this realization goes far beyond positive thinking. Yes, positive thoughts and emotions are associated with positive effects on our bodies, and negative thoughts and emotions are associated with negative effects. However, it isn't as simplistic as putting on a happy face to cure all your ills. Your thoughts, beliefs, and perceptions continually influence each other, and this is the platform with which you navigate through life.

Perceptions
↕   ↕
Thoughts ↔ Beliefs

Therefore, it would be wise for us to equip ourselves with thoughts, beliefs, and perceptions that would serve our health and wellbeing the most. The truth is that most of us are very unaware of how we think, never mind how we create the perceptions or beliefs that then govern our lives. One of the main reasons for this is that we spend the majority of each day operating from our subconscious mind, the part of the mind that contains that which is not in our direct awareness. We are creatures of habit and conditioning, operating all too often on autopilot, and it takes conscious work to change those patterns into those that will work for us rather than against us. Leading-edge scientist and author, Dr. Bruce Lipton, frequently writes and speaks about how our subconscious mind can easily sabotage our health and our very lives. Most of the programming we operate from as adults was picked up before the age of seven! Even if you are not yet open to the whole everything-is-energy paradigm, most of his research findings work on fundamental biology. Our blood chemistry is largely impacted by the chemicals emitted from our brain. Brain chemistry, via various neurotransmitters and hormones (messengers), adjusts the composition of the blood, based upon your perceptions of life. Recall from above that your perceptions influence how you think. Your thoughts, thereby, initiate various brain responses. You probably already know that high or regular concentrations of cortisol, commonly known as the stress hormone, can be extremely destructive.

As more people learn this, it is no surprise why we are seeing a continued popularity in the fields of personal development and mind-body techniques like meditation, emotional freedom technique (EFT), yoga, and all sorts of mindfulness practices. We need to become more conscious of our thoughts, beliefs, and perceptions, for it is only then that we can consciously begin to change them in favorable ways. As I already mentioned in this chapter, it is very easy to pick up mind viruses in a society that constantly bombards us with all sorts of information and stimuli. Basically, our minds are over-stimulated, and there is only so much information that can be processed effectively. This ties into the other reason why we operate so naturally on autopilot. Our brains are efficient and adaptable, so one of the easiest ways to cope with all the incoming information is to allow the subconscious mind to deal with it. This may or may not work to our advantage though. For example, if your mind continues to process the world as a scary, merciless, unjust, unpredictable, or dishonest place, your body will not flourish in good health. Likewise, if you live in a frequent state of fear, anger, regret, guilt, resentment, frustration, or inadequacy, you are putting yourself at a high risk of serious physical imbalance. We know today that we must manage the contents of our minds effectively if we are to have optimal health. As innovative thinkers, Carl Jung and his mentor, Sigmund Freud, taught, the psyche (mind) and the body are one, interconnected and constantly influencing each other. The mind moves the body. It can make us sick or well. It all depends on what is taking place at the mind level.

This brings us to another vital point that must be mentioned here to help you make this practical and easily applicable to your everyday life. Regardless of what happens in life, be it death, divorce, job loss, illness, financial loss, or any other possible trauma, it is not the actual event that is so destructive to our health. Rather, it is our perceptions about it; the perceptions are the source of our stress and suffering. This is why leading personal development experts like

Wayne Dyer, PhD echo the message, "Change your thoughts, change your life." My advice to you is to work on choosing your perceptions wisely and consciously, as much as possible. Rather than being unconsciously reactive, switch to responding with conscious mindfulness. Whether it is a news headline, office gossip, or a relationship challenge, the more you engage with your conscious mind, the more effective you will be in processing the event in the moment, rather than carrying residual stress with you forward. What is, is. What happened, happened and cannot be undone. It is only and always a matter of what are you going to do about it or in response to it that will determine its effect on you.

Either way, it is essential to take time to process events that you deem stressful or painful appropriately. Take a time-out, talk to a friend or therapist, spend some time in nature, get a massage, or reassess your priorities. Don't bottle things up or try to pretend they don't exist, for we know all too well today that suppressed or repressed emotions wreak havoc on our health. We literally need to get things off our minds, off our chests, and out of our bodies, lest we block the healthy flow of energy, which can manifest all sorts of conditions. In fact, trying to push away thoughts or emotions is a futile task. We may think we have done so on a conscious level, but they continue to fester on a subconscious level and even manifest in amplified ways. In 1987, Dr. Daniel Wegner, a psychology professor at Harvard University, conducted a study to demonstrate what most of us already know: In our efforts not to think about something, we actually end up having more thoughts about that topic.[3] This is known as the *rebound effect of thought suppression*, and hopefully, it will inspire us to take some serious mental inventory of what needs our conscious attention.

When we consider the process of disease manifestation, how well you understand its cause depends on how deep you go. Let's use the common cold as an example:

▸ **Physical:** At the uppermost surface level, its cause will be attributed to a virus.

▸ **Physical:** As we go deeper in our physical understanding, we learn that our immune system is capable of defending itself and repairing literally anything, but only if it is properly supported and maintained. Thus, we begin to understand the role of lifestyle factors like diet, sleep, and exercise and how they can strengthen or weaken the immune system, thereby preventing or allowing the manifestation of a cold.

▸ **Physical/Mental/Emotional:** Going even deeper in our understanding, we learn that a cold signifies that various stressors have been impacting us and gotten out of balance, as they have not been dealt with appropriately. This, in turn, translates to all sorts of imbalances on the physical level. A cold is usually one of the least-serious ways for our bodies to tell us that we need to take a break, reflect, and reassess our next steps.

▸ **Mental/Emotional:** Going deeper yet in our understanding, we learn that a cold manifests most easily as a result of congestion on a mental level, such as being overwhelmed. You are burning yourself out with your thoughts, which are not in alignment with your body and spirit. A cold can manifest in the head (sinus) region, the throat, or the chest or include all three, which holds further clues for us as to what our specific mind-body block may be.

This kind of analysis can be applied to every condition. Our bodies communicate with us all the time via numerous symptoms. Unfortunately, most of us are not listening. Instead, we try to interpret the body's symptoms as negative attributes that need to be done away with or silenced as soon as possible. While taking proper care to address your health is always important, it would be even more valuable to listen to our bodies and understand what the imbalances are trying to tell us. Have we been working too hard, not affording our bodies the physical or mental rest we require? Have we been holding some grudge or resentment from the past? Have we been caught up in worry or anxiety about the future? When the mind is out of balance with our inner being/soul/spirit, it eventually manifests, on some level, in the body. Think back to the last time you had an unpleasant exchange with someone. Your health can be impacted within minutes after such an event in an assortment of ways. For most people, it almost always includes some kind of digestive disturbance on the day of. Depending on how you perceived the situation, it might have manifested into an infection a few days later or even a more serious condition down the road.

Prevention starts with mindfulness. First, we need to process the event consciously and effectively; you will know this is effective when the event no longer triggers you in unpleasant ways. Second, we need to become more mindful of our thoughts, how and what we think about ourselves, first and foremost, others, and life situations, and choose more empowering, rather than disempowering thoughts, words and actions. Our thoughts are the precursors of our emotions. Yes, our emotions can influence our thoughts, but it all starts with the thoughts. As I have come to learn and now teach, our state of health (never mind our nutrition or lifestyle choices) always, always, always reflects the level of our self-love, self-worth, self-respect, and self-acceptance. Your body knows if you are being loving to it and yourself or not. We can fool our minds, but we cannot fool our bodies. The same is true in reverse as well: Our minds can fool us, tell us anything we wish to believe, try to downplay or negate that anything is wrong, but our bodies will never lie. If something manifests physically, you can bet there is a bigger mental-emotional imbalance that desperately requires attention.

When it comes to healing, its level of success, like that of prevention, will greatly depend on our willingness to visit what is hiding at the depths of our minds and work with it consciously. Each day, more and more conventional medical doctors are discovering the same conclusions as holistic health practitioners: Our success in healing has a multifactorial nature and should be addressed in a holistic way for the most effectiveness and sustainability. Changing our diet, detoxifying, and getting more physical exercise and proper rest are all important, but so are the changes that are needed at the mind level. We know hope, joy, gratitude, optimism, forgiveness, and other positive states contribute to better mental, emotional, and physical health and, consequently, healing.

One of the best books written on the subject of holistic healing comes from Dr. Elaine R. Ferguson, an integrative medical doctor. In *Superhealing: Engaging Your Mind, Body, and Spirit to Create Optimal Health and Wellbeing*, Dr. Ferguson presents research breakthroughs from different scientific fields, as well as her own professional experience on how to heal any imbalance and enjoy optimal wellbeing by involving the mind, body, and spirit. She explains the nature of the mind and body and their role in our health and healing but ultimately goes even further to address the role of the spirit, the core ingredient of the *superhealing* formula, and its many emotional manifestations. As she beautifully shares:

"The basis of our spiritual health and wellbeing is becoming one with life itself through the awareness of our inseparable connection to everyone and everything. It is escaping the unconsciously self-imposed constraints of our ego identity: the constricted individualized personality we have become through the portal of our culture's ideas of who we should be rather than the truth of who we are. Optimal health and wellbeing is not an end but a process, an adventure along the pathway of self-discovery."

Our health truly is in our hands, or perhaps our minds and spirits would be a better way of putting it. Wherever you are on your journey into optimal health, healing, and prevention, keep moving to keep uncovering the potential that awaits you. Remember that every journey begins with a single step. In order to effectively change the external conditions, we must change the internal: how we think and the perceptions and beliefs we choose to hold about ourselves, others, and all life. A drug or surgery may be needed on your journey of healing, but understand that while these may suppress a certain set of symptoms, if we don't make a serious change in our thinking, eating, and/or lifestyle habits, the body will express the imbalance in some other part or some other way. There is really no way around this. Depending on your personal background and understanding of health thus far, this information may elicit all sorts of thoughts and feelings. If this information is completely new to you, take time to process it and its many possibilities or, better yet, opportunities.

Yes, your diet will have a tremendous impact on your physical, mental, and emotional health. This is one of the reasons why it is often our best place to start on our journey into optimal wellbeing. Another reason is that it is tangible. If we begin by focusing on our minds, we may feel overwhelmed or uncertain of how to actually turn things around and break vicious patterns and years of negative thinking or self-talk. Not only will your food influence how your body works, but it will also influence how your brain and mind function. By taking steps to align your eating and lifestyle habits with the guidelines expressed in this book you engage in a powerfully practical approach that can help move you forward. As you continue to explore healthy eating and other lifestyle habits, you will naturally be drawn to go deeper in your personal journey and work effectively with the contents of your mind, which hold a critical piece of the optimal health, healing, and prevention puzzle. Without this piece, we will not be able to see or understand the full picture of our health. Both science and spirituality tell us today that meditation and mindfulness strengthen mental control. The more we feel conscious of and in control of our thoughts and our emotions, the more empowered we become to take effective action that is most suitable for our health and life.

To support you on this journey further, I have compiled a list of recommended books, films, and websites at the end of this book. Explore them as you feel called to do so. Know that the right support and resources are all around you; you only have to seek them and put into action the guidance they provide, as it best resonates with your inner being, values, and priorities.

Conclusion

We have come to the end of our journey together, have learned how to eat for optimal health and weight and to heal and prevent disease. The material presented in this book was meant to foster awareness, inspiration, motivation, and encouragement for your journey into superior nutrition and optimal health. Now it comes down to what you will choose to do with it, based on your personal vision. As mentioned in the introduction, the purpose of this book was not to revolutionize eating. Rather, it was written simply to remind us all of what many of us already know, to help guide you back to the path of properly supporting your health with food.

As we all know, one of the most commonly used excuses for not eating right is that we are too busy, that we simply don't have the time to visit a farmers' market, shop consciously, or prepare homemade meals from wholesome ingredients. But the time has come to release the excuses, to get honest, and to figure out our priorities and align our actions with them. Our health, weight, and wellbeing statistics—and perhaps your own poor quality of health—are sounding the alarm bells. What could be more important than feeding ourselves properly, being accountable for our health, and creating the state of health we desire? For many of us, taking a conscious approach to optimal health often coincides with taking a conscious reassessment of our daily lives. It is not our status, possessions, or our accomplishments that will bring deep-seated joy, fulfillment, or inner peace. Rather, we will gain this by living with meaning and purpose, harmony, and balance, in service and creativity, and in an optimally functioning body full of vigor and vitality, one that does not limit your personal daily expressions but enhances them!

Our personal expressions always create a ripple effect, regardless of what we are doing or being. We can improve the state of our world for ourselves and all others, or we can degrade it. We can be part of the solution or part of the problem. If you have children, regardless of their age, remember you will set the biggest example for them, and teach them about their relationship with food, health, and their bodies. You can integrate positive, healthy habits or ignite a lifetime of struggle with their health and weight. It is never too late to turn things around, for yourself or for them. Whether you are single, have a partner, or have a large family, each one of us must first be accountable for our personal choices that reflect the outcome we desire when it comes to our health and wellbeing. It is not about forcing anyone; rather, it is about providing the right tools, fostering a nurturing environment, and inspiring with our actions. We have more power at every turn than we often realize and it is my hope to bring you back to this empowered state of being.

Our society, culture, and healthcare system are shaped by our everyday choices. Therefore, choose wisely by choosing consciously. Every single action has a consequence, and repeated, similar actions turn into patterns, habits that can ultimately sabotage our health and our lives. Unconscious and conditioned destructive habits have carried us to the point where we are now. Awareness, coupled with conscious action, has the power to turn this all around. When we put poor-quality, nutrient-deficient, and toxin-filled foods into our bodies, we are creating bodies and health that reflect these very qualities. With this comes various biochemical imbalances, diseases, weight problems, loss of energy, vitality, and zest for life.

I know I don't have to tell you that obesity and weight problems are at epidemic rates. Lifestyle diseases are our number-one killers and destroyers of our quality of life. Our kids and young adults are continually exhibiting more of these same problems. Our babies are being born with or predisposed to a slew of various conditions at unprecedented levels. The prognosis is that this generation will not live as long as their parents if things continue as they are. What more do we need to motivate us into action? What more will it take to wake us up, to make us realize the value and importance of proper nutrition and health-conscious living?

I understand that it is not easy to make sense of proper nutrition today, particularly if one pays attention to the headlines, marketed products, and catchy diet fads. It can be easy, though, when we step out and away from the contradictory madness and consult our inner knowing. You will not find the answer to proper nutrition in the numbers game, the food guides, diets, and various food fads. It is not about moderation; as I mentioned before, eating everything in moderation is best if you want to have disease and weight problems in moderation. It is also not about excuses; just that one time is often a regular thing for most of us. Food author Michael Pollan has summarized it beautifully: "Eat food, not too much, mostly plants." This kind of simplicity is what we need more of today. As I will share again and again, eating was not and should not be trivial. It only becomes so when we get caught up in the fear, drama, and details created by industries that try to pull us in whatever direction suits their agenda and their profit margin.

If I speak with passion and certainty throughout this book it is mainly due to the fact that I have experienced for myself the power nutrition has on our optimal state of health and wellbeing. Based on my lifestyle choices, with superior nutrition being one of the key parts, I know firsthand that it is possible not to get sick, live lethargically, or age at the rate we've accepted today, as long as we properly address and support the balance of the mind, body, and spirit. While this is all great for me, I don't want to keep it to myself, I want to share this with others, in the hopes that it will help to alleviate so much unnecessary suffering. However, I cannot make your meals, change your habits, or feed you. Only you can do that for yourself and only when you decide to do so.

Poor health (physical, mental, and emotional) goes way beyond genetics, fate, karma, coincidence, or any isolated event. Poor health is directly related to our lifestyle habits and choices, namely our diets and how we feed ourselves. The sooner we recognize this and make the connection, the more we stand to benefit. You do not need to run out and read every nutrition book available or consult various nutritionists and specialists. All it takes is a more mindful, aware approach to eating. You were designed to know how to thrive, bring back that knowing.

Start at the grocery store, and walk among the numerous food packages consciously. It may be difficult to see the real food among all those pretty bags, boxes, and cans, but it is there. Colorful signs, claims, promises, ads, and labels are all around us, and convenience makes us want to forget what we know. This is why you need to make a decision about what you really want and stand strong, with conviction and determination. Once you gain enough momentum going for optimally healthy eating, the journey will only get easier and easier. Be conscious of your choices, and you are bound to be successful.

With your reusable bags full of real, fresh, natural food, go home and begin the creative process. As you've learned in this book, and as I'm happy to share with you in my other written and video resources, most wholesome, balanced meals can be prepared in 15 to 30 minutes and do not require fancy recipes or any culinary genius. It simply requires a conscious approach, some playfulness, and motivation. Make feeding yourself your number-one hobby. Fall in love with your food. Turn your kitchen into your own art studio, making your food and your meals your masterpieces. Get your creative juices flowing. Celebrate nourishing yourself properly and seeing your body respond accordingly. In the midst of it all, take the time to fall more in love with yourself, knowing that you *are* worth it and that you deserve to be nourished only with the very best.

It has been said over and over again and it is something most of us know first-hand: health truly is everything. Regardless of our successes or possessions, being in any debilitated state of health, whether it is a headache, chest infection, or cancer, decreases the quality of our lives. Our ability to enjoy all the beauty, variety, opportunity, and richness of life becomes severely limited. It only gets worse as we age; not because aging is meant to be hard or full of disease, but because the effects of a poor diet become compounded over many years and start to become increasingly obvious as we get older. The best news, though, is that our bodies are extremely resilient and it is never too late to nourish and support your body right. It may have taken years to get to a certain state of imbalance but the healing starts as soon as we begin the supportive process. When dietary excellence is combined with optimally healthy lifestyle habits and the power of the mind, the potential is unlimited!

I am 100 percent certain that our bodies were meant to last much longer than they do, and in a much better state. However, this journey is not about aiming for some state of immortality or trying to avoid death. The heart of it is about quality; living in the best state possible, savoring and enjoying every minute of this precious life experience, as long as we are here. I wish you an enjoyable and positively transformational journey and optimal health and wellbeing for each and every one of your days!

Resources

The following resources can provide further help on your journey of optimal health, healing, prevention, and nutritional excellence:

Books

1. Eat to Live by Dr. Joel Fuhrman

2. Whole: Rethinking the Science of Nutrition by Dr. T. Colin Campbell & Howard Jacobson

3. The China Study by Dr. T. Colin Campbell

4. Conscious Eating by Dr. Gabriel Cousens

5. The Biology of Belief by Dr. Bruce Lipton

6. Natural Health, Natural Medicine by Dr. Andrew Weil

7. The Acid-Alkaline Food Guide by Dr. Susan E. Brown & Larry Trivieri Jr.

8. Sugarettes by Dr. Scott Olson

9. Superhealing: Engaging Your Mind, Body and Spirit to Create Optimal Health and Wellbeing by Dr. Elaine R. Ferguson

10. Your Body's Telling You: Love Yourself! by Lise Bourbeau

11. Perfect Health the Natural Way by Mary-Ann Shearer

12. Your Natural Medicine Cabinet by Burke Lennihan

13. Better Health Through Natural Healing by Ross & Shea Tattler

14. The Thrive Diet by Brendan Brazier

15. In Defense of Food by Michael Pollan

16. **Virus of the Mind** by Richard Brodie

17. **Skinny Bitch** or **Skinny Bastard** by Rory Freedman & Kim Barnouin

Websites

1. **evolvingwellness.com** — Evita's article and recipe website

2. **healthytarian.com** — Evita's video recipe and tutorial website

3. **whfoods.org** — World's Healthiest Foods directory

4. **vegsource.com** — Vegan and vegetarian resources

5. **responsibletechnology.org** — Institute for Responsible Technology (GMO)

6. **tcolincampbell.org** — Dr. T. Colin Campbell (Plant-Based)

7. **heartattackproof.com** — Dr. Caldwell B. Esselstyn (Plant-Based)

8. **drfuhrman.com** — Dr. Joel Fuhrman (Plant-Based)

9. **nealbarnard.org** — Dr. Neal Barnard (Plant-Based)

10. **veganmd.org** — Dr. Michael Greger (Plant-Based)

11. **johnrobbins.info** — John Robbins (Plant-Based)

12. **doctorklaper.com** — Dr. Michael Klaper (Plant-Based)

13. **wellnessforum.com** — Dr. Pam Popper (Plant-Based)

14. **treeoflifecenterus.com** — Dr. Gabriel Cousens (Plant-Based)

15. **jeffnovick.com** — Jeff Novick (Dietitian, Plant-Based)

16. **brendadavisrd.com** — Brenda Davis (Dietitian, Plant-Based)

17. **theveganrd.com** — Ginny Kisch Messina (Dietitian, Plant-Based)

18. **choosingraw.com** — Gena Hamshaw (Raw, Plant-Based)

19. **berniesiegelmd.com** — Dr. Bernie Siegel (Mind-Body Healing)

20. **drnorthrup.com** — Dr. Christiane Northrup (Mind-Body Healing)

21. **drelaine.com** — Dr. Elaine Ferguson (Mind-Body Healing)

22. **lisebourbeau.com** — Lise Bourbeau (Mind-Body Healing)

Movies

1. Forks Over Knives — forksoverknives.com

2. Hungry for Change — hungryforchange.com

3. The Cure Is — thecureismovie.com

4. Food Inc. — foodincmovie.com

5. A Delicate Balance — adelicatebalance.com.au

6. PlanEAT — planeat.tv

7. Processed People — processedpeople.com

8. The Future of Food — thefutureoffood.com

9. Food Matters — foodmatters.tv

10. GMO OMG — gmofilm.com

11. Simply Raw — rawfor30days.com

12. Fresh — freshthemovie.com

13. In Organic We Trust — inorganicwetrust.org

14. Fat, Sick & Nearly Dead — fatsickandnearlydead.com

15. Farmageddon — farmageddonmovie.com

16. Peaceable Kingdom — peaceablekingdomfilm.org

17. You Can Heal Your Life — youcanhealyourlifemovie.com

References

Books

Adams, M. (2009). *Superfoods for optimum health: Chlorella and spirulina.* Truth Publishing. Retrieved from, http://www.naturalnews.com/specialreports/superfoods.pdf

Baroody, T. (1991). *Alkalize or die: Superior health through proper alkaline-acid balance.* Waynesville, NC: Eclectic.

Bourbeau, L. (2001). *Your body's telling you : Love yourself!: The most complete book on metaphysical causes of illnesses & diseases.* Bellefeuille, Québec: Éditions E.T.C.

Brodie, R. (2009). *Virus of the mind: The new science of the meme.* Carlsbad, Calif.: Hay House.

Brown, S., & Trivieri, L. (2013). *The acid alkaline food guide: A quick reference to foods & their effect on pH levels* (2nd ed.). New York: Square One.

Campbell, C. T., & Jacobson, H. (2013). *Whole: Rethinking the science of nutrition.* Dallas, TX.: BenBella Books.

Campbell, C. T., & Campbell, T. M. (2005). *The China study: The most comprehensive study of nutrition ever conducted and the startling implications for diet, weight loss and long-term health.* Dallas, TX: BenBella Books.

Cousens, G. (2000). *Conscious eating* (2nd ed.). Berkeley, CA: North Atlantic Books.

Cousens, G. (2005). *Spiritual nutrition: Six foundations for spiritual life and the awakening of Kundalini.* Berkeley, CA.: North Atlantic Books.

Esselstyn, C. (2007). *Prevent and reverse heart disease: The revolutionary, scientifically proven, nutrition-based cure.* New York: Avery.

Ferguson, E. (2013). *Superhealing: Engaging your mind, body, and spirit to create optimal health and well-being.* Deerfield Beach, FL: Health Communications.

Freedman, R., & Barnouin, K. (2009). *Skinny bastard: A kick-in-the-ass for real men who want to stop being fat and start getting buff.* Philadelphia: Running Press.

Fuhrman, J. (2011). *Eat to live: The amazing nutrient-rich program for fast and sustained weight loss* (Rev. ed.). New York: Little, Brown and Company.

Guerrero, A. (2005). *In balance for life.* Garden City Park, NY: Square One.

Lipton, B. (2007). *The biology of belief: Unleashing the power of consciousness, matter and miracles (Rev. ed.).* California: Hay House.

Logan, A. (2006). *The brain diet: The connection between nutrition, mental health, and intelligence.* Nashville, Tenn.: Cumberland House.

Lourie, B., & Smith, R. (2014). *Toxin toxout: Getting harmful chemicals out of our bodies and our world.* Toronto: Knopf Canada.

Olson, S. (2008). *Sugarettes: Sugar addiction and your health.* Charleston, S.C.: BookSurge Publishing.

Pollan, M. (2008). *In defense of food: An eater's manifesto.* New York: Penguin Press.

Selhub, E., & Logan, A. (2012). *Your brain on nature: The science of nature's influence on your health, happiness and vitality.* Mississauga, ON.: John Wiley & Sons Canada.

Weil, A. (2004). *Natural health, natural medicine: The complete guide to wellness and self-care for optimum health (Rev. ed.).* Boston, Mass.: Houghton Mifflin.

Young, R., & Young, S. (2002). *The pH miracle: Balance your diet, reclaim your health.* New York, NY: Warner Books.

Citations

Introduction

[1] Anand, P., Kunnumakara, A., Sundaram, C., Harikumar, K., Tharakan, S., Lai, O., Aggarwal, B., et al. (2008). Cancer is a preventable disease that requires major lifestyle changes. *Pharmaceutical Research, 259*(9), 2097-2116.

[2] David, A., & Zimmerman, M. (2010). Cancer: an old disease, a new disease or something in between? *Nature Reviews Cancer, 10,* 728-733.

[3] World Health Organization. (2011, April 1). Global status report on noncommunicable diseases 2010. Retrieved June 17, 2011, from http://www.who.int/nmh/publications/ncd_report2010/en/World Health Organization.

Chapter 1

[1] Langford, N., & Ferner, R. (1999). Toxicity of mercury. *Journal of Human Hypertension, 13*(10), 651-656.

[2] Jones, O., Maguire, M., & Griffin, J. (2008). Environmental pollution and diabetes: A neglected association. *The Lancet, 26*(371), 287-288.

Chapter 2

[1] De la Monte, S., Neusner, A., Chu, J., & Lawton, M. (2009). Epidemilogical trends strongly suggest exposures as etiologic agents in the pathogenesis of sporadic Alzheimer's disease, Diabetes Mellitus, and non-alcoholic Steatohepatitis. *The Journal of Alzheimer's Disease,* 17(3), 519-529.

[2] Pobel, D., Riboli, E., Cornée, J., Hémon, B., & Guyader, M. (1995). Nitrosamine, nitrate and nitrite in relation to gastric cancer: A case-control study in Marseille, France. *European Journal of Epidemiology,* 11(1), 67-73.

[3] American Heart Association. (2014, May 19). Frequently asked questions (FAQs) about sodium. Retrieved June 6, 2014, from http://www.heart.org/HEARTORG/GettingHealthy/NutritionCenter/HealthyEating/Frequently-Asked-Questions-FAQs-About-Sodium_UCM_306840_Article.jsp.

[4] Fuhrman, J. (2013, March 17). Salt drives autoimmune disease? *Dr. Fuhrman's Disease Proof.* Retrieved June 6, 2014, from http://www.diseaseproof.com/archives/autoimmune-diseases-salt-drives-autoimmune-disease.html.

Chapter 3

[1] Dunn, R. (2012, July 23). Human ancestors were nearly all vegetarians. *Scientific American.* Retrieved June 7, 2014, from http://blogs.scientificamerican.com/guest-blog/2012/07/23/human-ancestors-were-nearly-all-vegetarians/

[2] Zuk, M. (2009, January 19). The evolutionary search for our perfect past. *The New York Times.* Retrieved June 7, 2014, from http://www.nytimes.com/2009/01/20/health/views/20essa.html?_r=0

[3] Dunn, R. (2012, August 2). How to eat like a chimpanzee. *Scientific American.* Retrieved June 7, 2014, http://blogs.scientificamerican.com/guest-blog/2012/08/02/how-to-eat-like-a-chimpanzee/

[4] Ibid.

Chapter 4

[1] Frassetto, L., Morris, R., Sellmeyer, D., Todd, K., & Sebastian, A. (2001). Diet, evolution and aging--the pathophysiologic effects of the post-agricultural inversion of the potassium-to-sodium and base-to-chloride ratios in the human diet. *European Journal of Nutrition,* 40(5), 200-13.

[2] Vormann, J. (2006, September). 2nd International acid-base symposium 2006. *Saure Basen Forum.* Retrieved June 10, 2014, from http://www.saeure-basen-forum.de/index.php/en/2nd-int-acid-base-symposium

[3] Vormann, J., & Remer, T. (2008). Dietary, metabolic, physiologic, and disease-related aspects of acid-base balance: foreword to the contributions of the second international acid-base symposium. *The Journal of Nutrition*, 138(2), 413S-414S.

[4] Schwalfenberg, G. (2012). The alkaline diet: Is there evidence that an alkaline pH diet benefits health? *Journal of Environmental and Public Health*, 2012, 1-7.

[5] Ibid [1]

Chapter 5

[1] Steinmetz, K., & Potter, J. (1996). Vegetables, fruit, and cancer prevention: A review. *Journal of the American Dietetic Association*, 96(10), 1027–1039.

[2] Dunn, R. (2012, August 27). The hidden truths about calories. *Scientific American*. Retrieved July 2, 2014, http://blogs.scientificamerican.com/guest-blog/2012/08/27/the-hidden-truths-about-calories/

[3] Uribarri, J., Cai, W., Sandu, O., Peppa, M., Goldberg, T., & Vlassara, H. (2005). Diet-derived advanced glycation end products are major contributors to the body's AGE pool and induce inflammation in healthy subjects. *Annals of the New York Academy of Sciences*, 1043, 461-466.

[4] Luevano-Contreras, C., & Chapman-Novakofski, K. (2010). Dietary advanced glycation end products and aging. *Nutrients*, 2, 1247-1265.

[5] Chappell, Mary Margaret. (n.d.). High cooking temperature and inflammation. *Arthritis Foundation*. Retrieved July 3, 2014, from http://www.arthritistoday.org/what-you-can-do/eating-well/arthritis-diet/cooking-temperature-inflammation.php

Chapter 6

[1] Seralini, G., Mesnage, R., Clair, E., Gress, S., Spiroux de Vendomois, J., & Cellier, D. (2011). Genetically modified crops safety assessments: Present limits and possible improvements. *Environmental Sciences Europe*, 23(10). Retrieved July 4, 2014, from http://www.enveurope.com/content/23/1/10

[2] Asami, D., Hong, Y., Barrett, D., & Mitchell, A. (2003). Comparison of the total phenolic and ascorbic acid content of freeze-dried and air-dried marionberry, strawberry, and corn grown using conventional, organic, and sustainable agricultural practices. *Journal of Agricultural and Food Chemistry*, 51(5), 1237-1241.

[3] The Benefits of Organic Agriculture: Review of Scientific Research & Studies. (n.d.). Retrieved July 5, 2014, from http://natturan.is/site_media/uploads/tun_benefits_of_oa.pdf

[4] Reganold, J., Andrews, P., Reeve, J., Carpenter-Boggs, L., Schadt, C., Alldredge, J., et al. (2010). Fruit and soil quality of organic and conventional strawberry agroecosystems. *PLoS ONE*, 5(9), E12346-E12346.

Chapter 8

[1] Herbert, V. (1988). Vitamin B12: Plant sources, requirements and assay. *American Journal of Clinical Nutrition*, 48, 852-858.

[2] Ibid.

Chapter 10

[1] World's Healthiest Foods. (n.d.). Whole grains: Oats. *World's Healthiest Foods.* Retrieved May 20, 2014, http://www.whfoods.com/genpage.php?tname=foodspice&dbid=54

Chapter 12

[1] Bilsborough, S., & Mann, N. (2006). A review of issues of dietary protein intake in humans. *International Journal of Sport Nutrition and Exercise Metabolism*, 16(2), 129-52.

[2] Agriculture Fact Book 2001-2002. (2003, March 1). *U.S. Department of Agriculture.* Retrieved May 25, 2014, from http://www.usda.gov/factbook/2002factbook.pdf

[3] Hamershlag, K. (2011). Report - 2011 Meat Eaters Guide | Meat and your Health. *Environmental Working Group.* Retrieved May 27, 2014, from http://www.ewg.org/meateatersguide/a-meat-eaters-guide-to-climate-change-health-what-you-eat-matters/meat-and-your-health/

[4] Wang, Y., & Beydoun, M. (2009). Meat consumption is associated with obesity and central obesity among U.S. adults. *International Journal of Obesity*, 33(6), 621-628.

[5] Campbell, T., & Campbell, T. (2005). The China study: The most comprehensive study of nutrition ever conducted and the startling implications for diet, weight loss and long-term health. Dallas, Tex.: BenBella Books.

[6] Koeth, R., Wang, Z., Levison, B., et al. (2013). Intestinal microbiota metabolism of L-carnitine, a nutrient in red meat, promotes atherosclerosis. *Nature Medicine*, 19, 576-585.

[7] Ibid [5].

Chapter 13

[1] Halldorsson, T., Strom, M., Petersen, S., & Olsen, S. (2010). Intake of artificially sweetened soft drinks and risk of preterm delivery: A prospective cohort study in 59,334 Danish pregnant women. *American Journal of Clinical Nutrition*, 92(3), 626-633.

[2] Bray, G. (2007). How bad is fructose? *American Journal of Clinical Nutrition*, 86(4), 895-896.

[3] Smith-Warner, S., Spiegelman, D., Shiaw-Shyuan, Y., et al. (1998). Alcohol and breast cancer in women: A pooled analysis of cohort studies. *JAMA: The Journal of the American Medical Association*, 279(7), 535-540.

[4] Mayo Clinic Staff. (n.d.) Red wine and resveratrol: Good for your heart?.*Mayo Clinic.* Retrieved March 4, 2011, from http://www.mayoclinic.com/health/red-wine/ HB00089

Chapter 14

[1] Bray, G., Nielsen, S., & Popkin, B. (2004). Consumption of high-fructose corn syrup in beverages may play a role in the epidemic of obesity. *American Journal of Clinical Nutrition*, 79(4), 537-543.

[2] Al-shahib, W., & Marshall, R. (2003). The fruit of the date palm: Its possible use as the best food for the future? *International Journal of Food Sciences and Nutrition*, 54(4), 247-259.

[3] Boston University Medical Center. (2013, April 22). Mushrooms can provide as much vitamin D as supplements. *ScienceDaily*. Retrieved June 16, 2014 from www.sciencedaily.com/releases/2013/04/130422132801.htm.

[4] Koyyalamudi, S., Jeong, S., Cho, K., & Pang, G. (2009). Vitamin B12 is the active corrinoid produced in cultivated white button mushrooms (Agaricus bisporus). *Journal of Agricultural and Food Chemistry*, 57(14), 6327-6333.

[5] Gan, C., Nurul, A., & Asmah, R. (2013). Antioxidant analysis of different types of edible mushrooms (Agaricus bisporous and Agaricus brasiliensis). *International Food Research Journal*, 20(3), 1095-1102.

[6] Witkowska, A., Zujko, M., & Mironczuk-Chodakowska, I. (2011). Comparative study of wild edible mushrooms as sources of antioxidants. *International Journal of Medicinal Mushrooms*, 13(4), 335-341.

[7] Ferreira, I., Barros, L., & Abreu, R. (2009). Antioxidants in wild mushrooms. *Current Medicinal Chemistry*, 16(12), 1543-1560.

Chapter 16

[1] Sloan, E., & Adams Hutt, C. (2013, October 1). Reading the compass: Up-and-coming market trends. *Nutraceuticals World*. Retrieved December 18, 2013, from http:// www.nutraceuticalsworld.com/issues/2013-10/view_features/reading-the-compass-up-and-coming-market-trends/

[2] Gahche, J., Bailey, R., Burt, V., & Hughes, J. (2011, April 13). Dietary Supplement Use Among U.S. Adults Has Increased Since NHANES III (1988-1994). *Centers for Disease Control and Prevention*. Retrieved July 12, 2011, from http:// www.cdc.gov/nchs/data/databriefs/db61.htm

[3] Eberhardt, M., Liu, R., & Lee, C. (2000). Antioxidant activity of fresh apples. *Nature*, 405(6789), 903-904.

[4] Brasky, T., Darke, A., Song, X., Tangen, C., Goodman, P., Thompson, I., Kristal, A., et al. (2013). Plasma phospholipid fatty acids and prostate cancer risk in the SELECT trial. *Journal of the National Cancer Institute*, 105(15), 1132-1141.

[5] Roncaglioni, M., Tombesi, M., Avanzini, F., Barlera, S., Caimi, V., Longoni, P., et al. (2013). N–3 fatty acids in patients with multiple cardiovascular risk factors. *New England Journal of Medicine*, 368(19), 1800-1808.

[6] Chalmers, A., & Martinsen, B. (2013, July 14). The rancid truth about omega-3 fish oil facts on freshness, fish oil and your health. *Omega 3 Innovations*. Retrieved December 28, 2013, from http://ww1.prweb.com/prfiles/2013/07/14/10927185/rancidtruth.pdf

[7] Omega-3 och Hälsa. (n.d.). Omega-3 in Vegetarian Food? *Omega-3 och Hälsa*. Retrieved March 10, 2011, from http://www.omega-3.se/en/vegetarian.html

[8] Simopoulos, A. (2008). The omega-6/omega-3 fatty acid ratio, genetic variation, and cardiovascular disease. *Asia Pacific Journal of Clinical Nutrition*, 17(Suppl 1), 131-134.

Chapter 18

[1] Environmental Working Group. (2013, May). Canaries in the kitchen: Heated pans get toxic in minutes. *Environmental Working Group*. Retrieved June 20 2014, from http://www.ewg.org/research/canaries-kitchen/heated-pans-get-toxic-minutes

[2] Gray, Kurt. (2012). The power of good intentions: Perceived benevolence soothes pain, increases pleasure, and improves taste." *Social Psychological and Personality Science, 3(5)*, 639-645.

Chapter 19

[1] Foster-Schubert, K., Alfano, C., Duggan, C., Xiao, L., Campbell, K., Kong, A., Mctiernan, A., et al. (2012). Effect of diet and exercise, alone or combined, on weight and body composition in overweight-to-obese postmenopausal women. *Obesity*, 20(8), 1628–1638.

[2] Mcferran, B., & Mukhopadhyay, A. (2013). Lay theories of obesity predict actual body mass. *Psychological Science*, 24(8), 1428-1436.

[3] Myers, J. (2003). Exercise and cardiovascular health. *Circulation*, 107(1), E2-E5.

[4] Sharma, A., Madaan, V., & Petty, F. (2006). Exercise for mental health. *Journal of Clinical Psychiatry*, 8(2), 106.

[5] Jones, J. (2013, December 19). In U.S., 40% Get Less Than Recommended Amount of Sleep. Retrieved June 29, 2014, from http://www.gallup.com/poll/166553/less-recommended-amount-sleep.aspx

[6] Insufficient Sleep Is a Public Health Epidemic. (2014, January 13). *Centers for Disease Control and Prevention*. Retrieved June 29, 2014, from http://www.cdc.gov/features/dssleep/

[7] National Sleep Foundation. (n.d.). How Much Sleep Do We Really Need? *National Sleep Foundation*. Retrieved June 29, 2014, from http://sleepfoundation.org/how-sleep-works/how-much-sleep-do-we-really-need

[8] Berman, M., Jonides, J., & Kaplan, S. (2008). The cognitive benefits of interacting with nature. *Psychological Science*, 19(12), 1207-1212.

[9] University of Oxford. (2014, May 22). Fruit flies show mark of intelligence in thinking before they act, study suggests. *ScienceDaily*. Retrieved June 30, 2014 from www.sciencedaily.com/releases/2014/05/140522141426.htm

[10] National Center for Complementary and Alternative Medicine. (2010, June 1). Meditation: An Introduction. *National Institutes of Health*. Retrieved June 30, 2014, from http://nccam.nih.gov/health/meditation/overview.htm

Chapter 20

[1] Gómez-Pinilla, F. (2008). Brain foods: The effects of nutrients on brain function. *Nature Reviews Neuroscience*, 9(7), 568-578.

[2] Sánchez-Villegas, A., Toledo, E., Irala, J., Ruiz-Canela, M., Pla-Vidal, J., & Martínez-González, M. (2012). Fast-food and commercial baked goods consumption and the risk of depression. *Public Health Nutrition*, 15(3), 424-432.

[3] Wegner, D., Schneider, D., Carter, S., & White, T. (1987). Paradoxical effects of thought suppression. *Journal of Personality and Social Psychology*, 53(1), 5-13.

About the Author

Evita Ochel B.Sc, B.Ed, CHN

Evita is a consciousness expansion teacher, writer, speaker, and Web TV host. She holds an honors bachelor of science degree in the areas of biology and psychology and a bachelor of education degree in the areas of science and mathematics. She is a natural health expert, certified holistic nutritionist, and certified yoga teacher.

Her passion for teaching and empowering others to live the highest quality of life is reflected in all of her creative endeavors: written and video resources, teaching platforms, and events. She taught high school science for seven years, and since 2009, she has been teaching worldwide, online and in-person, providing guidance and resources for all areas of the mind, body, and spirit. She is the author and creator of seven websites and two video networks that feature hundreds of essays, articles, reviews, recipes, videos, and photographs. Along her personal journey into optimal wellness, she created the *Healthytarian* lifestyle, based on *Fresh Thinking, Smart Eating,* and *Mindful Living.*

Evita prioritizes living in balance, reverence, and with utmost compassion for self, others, and all parts of nature. Aside from reading, writing, and researching, she spends a lot of time in nature, hiking, canoeing, growing her own food, foraging for wild foods, and simply being.

For more information about Evita or her work, visit www.EvitaOchel.com

Made in the USA
San Bernardino, CA
04 December 2014